MARIJUANA FOR EVERYBODY!

High Times

presents

MARIJUANA FOR EVERYBODY!

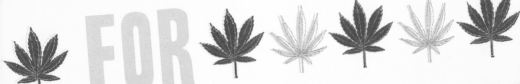

The DEFINITIVE GUIDE to Getting High, Feeling Good, and Having Fun ❦ Elise McDonough

CHRONICLE BOOKS

SAN FRANCISCO

Contents

Text copyright © 2014 by
Trans-High Corporation.
Illustrations copyright © 2014 by
Toby Triumph.

High Times and Cannabis Cup are
trademarks of the Trans-High Corporation
and are used with permission.

Library of Congress Cataloging-in-
Publication Data is available.

ISBN: 978-1-4521-2888-7

Manufactured in China

Designed by Hillary Caudle

10 9 8 7 6 5 4 3 2 1

Chronicle Books LLC
680 Second Street
San Francisco, CA 94107
www.chroniclebooks.com

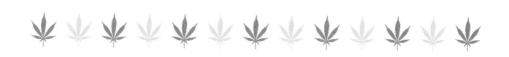

Introduction

Tremendous strides have been made in recent years toward legalizing, regulating, and retailing cannabis, making the once demonized weed more safely accessible to millions of people from sea to shining THC. Many of them experience tremendous healing and relief via the plant's unique medicinal benefits, while others simply enjoy indulging in a far safer method of altering their consciousness than mere alcohol can provide.

Public opinion regarding marijuana has at last reached a "spliffing point." At the time of writing, a majority of Americans favor legalization, and dozens of states—most notably Washington and Colorado—have variously legalized medical marijuana, decriminalized possession, or legalized it outright for adult use, with still more states moving in that direction.

Naturally we at *High Times* magazine take great pleasure in seeing marijuana finally going mainstream and getting its due. For forty years, we've advocated for the right of adults to responsibly use cannabis, bringing our readers the kind of in-depth pot reporting that nobody else can even attempt.

And so, as a fragrant wind of change steadily blows us toward ever greater acceptance of pot and pot smokers, it's high time that we share what we've learned from real experts and aficionados about the best ways to get high, feel good, and have fun with this amazing all-natural plant.

Marijuana for Everybody! collects this wisdom in a fun, accessible, authoritative handbook to one of life's greatest and most misunderstood natural resources. Here you'll find time-tested wisdom from growers, connoisseurs, activists, advocates, scientists, doctors, politicians, philosophers, and cannabis celebrities in the know, plus answers to burning questions and hand-selected, choice nuggets from the venerable marijuana magazine's four decades of publishing, all designed to guide new initiates and seasoned heads alike through the myriad ways marijuana brings joy and relief to millions while serving as the sacred sacrament of an ascendant cannabis culture.

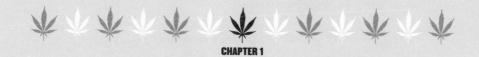

the
How and Why
of
Getting High

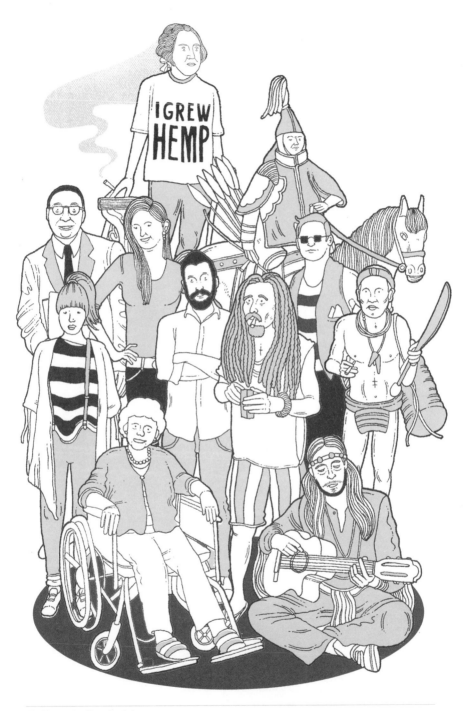

Marijuana for Everybody!

History of Cannabis

OUR LITTLE GREEN FRIEND

In the popular consciousness, marijuana burst onto the scene in a major way in the 1960s, as if America's hippie generation somehow discovered the amazing properties of this magnificent plant all on their own. But what most squares didn't realize back then, and still don't know today, is that the benevolent botanical called *Cannabis sativa* actually first befriended mankind way back at the dawn of pre-history, when the herb's many utilitarian functions as a fiber, food, medicine, and spiritual aid helped spark the development of ancient cultures.

> **"What is a weed? A plant whose virtues have not yet been discovered."**
>
> RALPH WALDO EMERSON

PREHISTORIC POT

Stoner scholars trace the likely origin of the cannabis plant to the original "Emerald Triangle" formed by Samarkand, the Hindu Kush mountains, and the Tien Shan mountains—a landmass encompassing the modern-day countries of Tajikistan, Kyrgyzstan, and Uzbekistan.

As far back as 6000 B.C.E., ancient Chinese peoples used highly nutritious cannabis seeds as a food source, while the earliest evidence of the plant's use as a fiber crop dates to Neolithic times over twelve thousand years ago, when hemp ropes were used to make decorative impressions into pottery. A well-preserved site in Zhejiang province yielded several examples of hemp textiles from 4000 B.C.E., while warriors in Shantung province circa 2300 B.C.E. wore armor sewn together by strong hemp cords—one of the earliest examples of hemp's role as a strategically vital natural resource and key to military supremacy.

Archeologists have recently made discoveries proving that people used cannabis as fiber and medicine much earlier in history than previously believed. A well-preserved Neolithic site called Çatalhöyük, located in Turkey, contained a nine-thousand-year-old piece of hemp cloth. Cannabis pollen was present in a 4,200-year-old gravesite near the town of Hattemer-broek, in the Netherland's largest province of Gelderland, the discovery of which occurred during construction of the Hanzelijn railway, and showed that certain among the Dutch appreciated getting stoned long before the first Amsterdam coffeeshop opened. The tombs also contained meadowsweet, another medicinal plant with pain relieving and fever-reducing properties, leading archaeologists to conclude that their occupant must have been ill before death. This key bit of evidence establishes medicinal use of cannabis in Europe very early in human history.

Cannabis seeds were eagerly traded as a food, fiber, and medicine, spreading this commodity all over the world. Nutritious seeds were also favored by many migratory birds that aided in the propagation of the species, another factor that helps explain the herb's rapid spread to almost every corner of the globe.

MEDICINE MAN

Emperor Shen Nung, the true O.G. of traditional Chinese medicine, who lived sometime between 2700 and 2300 B.C.E. and is still a revered figure, called cannabis one of the "Supreme Elixirs of Immortality." His *Pen Ts'ao Ching*, or "Great Herbal," is one of the oldest known pharmacopoeias, compiled from Shen's writings sometime in the first or second century B.C.E. In it, Shen documents the many medicinal uses of cannabis for the first time, recommending it to treat over one hundred different maladies, from gout and rheumatism to absentmindedness. In folk medicine, marijuana was used in the form of a tea or edible extract, and it would have been psychoactive to varying degrees. Shen Nung also makes note of the superior healing power of cultivating only female cannabis plants for their medicinal properties. (Seedless female flowers, now known as *sinsemilla*, contain more psychoactive resin than seeded plants.)

Mention was made of the psycho-active properties of cannabis in this early pharmacopoeia, but Shen Nung considered the medicinal uses more important. Other ancient peoples did use cannabis for its visionary properties, since the mystical village shaman was also a healer. The 2008 discovery of the mummified remains of a Gushi shaman who roamed the plains of Northwestern China over 2,700 years show that there were some who had already "turned on and tuned in."

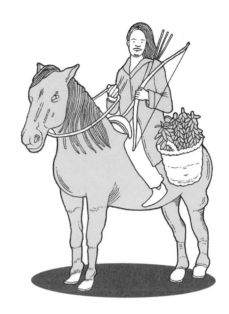

Called "Cherchen man," the mummy had blond hair and blue eyes, stood over six feet tall, and was approximately forty-five years old

Cherchen man, with stash.

when he died. Inside his tomb, besides other high-value items like bridles, brilliantly woven cloth, archery gear, and a harp, archeologists discovered almost two pounds of highly potent cannabis, a psychoactive head stash most likely meant for use in the afterlife. Experts speculate that this ancient spiritual guide must have eaten the cannabis (it would need preparation beforehand) or inhaled it over a burning fire, since no smoking tools accompanied the herb.

REEFER AND RELIGION

In Central Asia, around 2000 B.C.E., wandering Aryan and Muslim tribes spread cannabis from their homelands to the Indian Himalayas, Persia, and the Middle East, where it was enthusiastically embraced as a multipurpose resource. The Hindus even integrated the plant into their religion, calling it "a gift to the world from the god Shiva." The Sanskrit word for this wonderful new plant was *canna*, meaning "cane." The Greeks would later call it *Kannabis*, providing the inspiration for the modern scientific name *Cannabis sativa*, as taxonomist Carolus Linnaeus dubbed the plant in 1753.

Smelling just as sweet no matter what its name, this weedy camp follower steadily adapted to new and widely varying climates as it spread, splitting into several distinct subspecies along the way. In the colder climates of northern Europe, the fibrous hemp plant established itself as *ruderalis*, while more psychoactive *sativa* strains developed in the warmer southern climates of India, Persia, the Middle East, and Africa. Eventually, shrubby Afghani varieties became distinct enough from the tall, willowy plants in Asia or Europe to distinguish them as *Cannabis indica*, a subspecies with wide leaves and resistance to chilly mountain weather that was selectively bred to make hashish.

As various civilizations interacted with the plant, they would carry over and sometimes devise new uses for their favorite flora. Intentional inhalation of cannabis smoke for the purpose of getting high didn't become commonplace until after tobacco was introduced to the Old World in the early sixteenth century. For most of ancient history, the plant was used in topical applications or processed into hashish and eaten. However, the Scythian descendants of nomadic Aryans stumbled upon inhaling cannabis smoke for its euphoric qualities around 700 to 300 B.C.E. This earliest "hot boxing" happened when Scythians threw *canna* branches into bonfires they trapped under tents in order to form a psychedelic sweat lodge that made them "howl with pleasure." The practice was soon imitated in Africa after traders introduced cannabis from the Middle East, along with Portuguese sailors from India who facilitated its adoption on the eastern coast.

Called *dagga* and regarded as a tool of spiritual insight, the plant was thrown onto bonfires and used in rituals along with drumming, singing, and dancing by the Pygmies, Zulus, and Hottentots. Shamans in Africa revered cannabis as a sacred plant, and believed that the changes in consciousness associated with its use could reveal hidden knowledge and the power to heal.

Prior to the formation of the Roman Catholic Church, a form of Christianity was practiced in Ethiopia with cannabis as a central sacrament. This explains why the earliest known ceramic bongs were recovered in a cave in Ethiopia and date to 1320. And even today, the Ethiopian Zion Coptic Church performs a cannabis-based Eucharist ritual traced back to their earliest ancestors.

The Old Testament's recipe for "holy anointing oil," for example, included infusing the oil with large amounts of an ingredient called "kanna-bosm"—also known as cannabis—which is Aramaic for "fragrant cane."

WAS JESUS A STONER?

🌿🌿🌿🌿🌿🌿🌿🌿🌿🌿

In his controversial 2003 article for *High Times*, "Was Jesus a Stoner?," religious scholar Chris Bennett made a compelling case that the scientific basis for the healing miracles described in the Bible are likely due to "kanna-bosm."

"This holy anointing oil, as described in the original Hebrew version of the recipe in Exodus (30:22-23), contained over six pounds of kanna-bosm," Bennett explains, "a substance identified by respected etymologists, linguists, anthropologists, botanists, and other researchers as cannabis, extracted into about six quarts of olive oil, along with a variety of other fragrant herbs." Such a high concentration of cannabis would have rendered this oil potently psychoactive. Bennett notes that in the ancient world, people thought diseases like epilepsy were caused by demonic possession, and so if an epileptic was cured, this "miraculous healing" was considered to be a heroic feat on par with an exorcism. And cannabis is in fact highly effective in treating many of the ailments healed by Jesus, such as skin diseases (Matthew 8, 10, 11; Mark 1; Luke 5, 7, 17), eye problems (John 9: 6-15), and menstrual problems (Luke 8:43-48).

"Christ" is the Greek translation of the Hebrew "Messiah," a term best translated into English as "anointed one." According to the Bible, Jesus anointed his twelve apostles and instructed them to go out into the world and anoint others. "And they cast out many devils, and anointed with oil many that were sick, and healed them." (Mark 6:13) Gnostic accounts excluded from Roman Catholic Church canon include *The Acts of Peter and the Twelve Apostles*, which predates the New Testament, describing Jesus as bestowing a box of "unguent" (oil) and a "pouch full of medicine" on his followers and telling them to minister to the sick. Christ taught his followers to heal "the bodies first" before they could "heal the heart."

Although many Gnostic works were destroyed as heresy, Bennett finds that "The surviving Gnostic descriptions of the effects of the anointing rite make it very clear that the holy oil had intense psychoactive properties that prepared the recipient for entrance into 'unfading bliss.'"

At the time Jesus and his apostles supposedly used cannabis for its healing properties (see "Was Jesus a Stoner?"), the "fragrant cane" was already a well-established traditional folk remedy throughout the Middle East, as confirmed by modern archeological evidence. Ancient Assyrians used cannabis smoke to cure arthritis, which they called "the poison of all limbs." And cannabis ash was discovered in the Jerusalem tomb of a young girl who died in childbirth around the fourth century, presumably kept on hand as an herbal remedy to ease the pain of labor and speed delivery.

Many other religions were also sparked by psychedelic experiences and revelations. This phenomenon inspired a group of ethnobotanists and mythological scholars to coin the word *entheogen* in 1979 to describe certain psychoactive plants used in a shamanic or ritualized context, in order to "generate the divine within," and inspire spiritual insight. It's believed that the Zoroastrians of ancient Persia pioneered the religious use of cannabis, which their priest class adopted as a holy sacrament. The three Magi who attended the birth of Christ—famously bringing gold, frankincense, and myrrh—were Zoroastrians, whose mystical traditions inspired the word *magic,* for these Magi were seen as having otherworldly powers. The Zoroastrians later converted to Islam, forming a mystical sect known as the Sufis, who believe that cannabis brings divine revelation and oneness with Allah.

By the eleventh century, hashish eating became widespread throughout Arabia, with early texts calling cannabis by names like *shrub of emotion, shrub of understanding, peace of mind, branches of bliss,* and *thought morsel.* The oldest Arabic monograph on hashish, called *Zahr al-'arish fi tahrim al-hashish,* dates to the thirteenth century. Around the same time, Sufis filled the streets of nearby Cairo, bringing with them copious amounts of hashish and collectively cultivating an urban ganja garden in a park known as Cafour. The Egyptian authorities didn't find the ongoing pot party too groovy, however, and launched one of history's first drug wars to push them out in 1253.

After the Cafour gardens were burned, cannabis production moved outside the city, but the persecution did not end. Cannabis farmers continued to face execution, while hashish eaters had their teeth yanked out as punishment.

In Europe, the growing power of the Roman Catholic Church led to violent suppression of nature-worshipping pagan tribes and their rituals. Mystic folk healers who used cannabis and other plants to create medicinal "potions" were tortured or killed, driving the use of cannabis deep underground. From the Middle Ages to the nineteenth century, friends of cannabis had to hide, so little mention of their activities can be found in the historical record.

A SOURCE OF HAPPINESS

In India, the religious use of *gunjah* (a.k.a. ganja) began sometime around 2000 B.C.E. India also served as one of the earliest centers for hashish production, which at the time meant resin hand-rubbed from plants and rolled into small balls called *charas* that could be eaten or smoked out of a chillum.

According to the sacred Hindu texts called The Vedas, *gunjah*—one of five sacred plants—was "a source of happiness" that would "release us from anxiety." Associated with the Lord Shiva, *gunjah* most often appeared as part of a refreshing drink called bhang, made from milk, pounded nuts, ginger, and garam masala (see "Shiva's *Sativa* Bhang" recipe on page 142).

India's most renowned cannabis enthusiasts—ascetics known as *sadhus*—shun material life and live simply in the forests, growing long beards and wearing only loincloths or ragged clothing, while striving for spiritual freedom and seeking divinity by fasting, keeping celibate, and smoking *gunjah* and *charas*. It's believed that using bhang helps a *sadhu* honor Shiva, who was legendarily always high on cannabis. Bhang is still used at festivals such as Holi, where celebrants douse themselves in colored pigments that add to the sensual and psychedelic nature of the festivities.

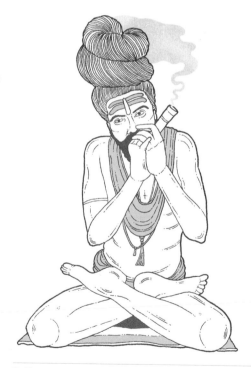

Sadhu smoking from a chillum.

EMPIRE AND EXPLORATION

The Roman Empire, which required massive amounts of hemp for its huge military, devoted entire cities like Ephesus and Mylasa to the industry of cannabis cultivation. By the fifteenth century, use of hemp for textiles and rope was commonplace throughout Europe. To increase the value of the hemp harvest and the height of their plants, peasants ritualistically jumped over (nonpsychoactive) bonfires and danced on rooftops.

Eventually hemp played a central role in the world's geopolitical balance of power, much as crude oil reserves do today. With sturdy hemp cords and canvas enabling sailing ships to travel into rough waters far from the coasts, a new era of powerful navies and far-flung exploration took hold. In fact, the first Old World visitors to the continent of North America, the Vikings, used hemp sails and ropes to make the arduous journey, and even carried hemp seeds with them in case of shipwreck. Then the Dutch began using their iconic windmills to crush tough, fibrous hemp stalks, a highly efficient processing method that soon enabled them to establish seafaring trade routes as far away as Asia.

> "Make the most of the Indian hemp seed, and sow it everywhere!"
>
> GEORGE WASHINGTON

Seeking to crack the Dutch domination of the high seas, the English secured hemp from Russia, a steady supply that helped propel their exploration of the recently discovered New World. When the Europeans at last reached North America, they found hemp crops already thriving. Archaeological evidence actually traces the continent's earliest known hemp to structures built by the Hopewell Mound Builders, who lived circa 400 B.C.E. in modern-day Ohio. In fact, ancient peoples throughout the Americas apparently used hemp for many purposes, although it's not clear how the plant originally arrived and took root. After the influx of colonists, the prerevolutionary American hemp crop became so incredibly vital that farmers were required to grow a certain acreage by law. Early American revolutionaries like George Washington then realized that by keeping the

> "Hemp is of first necessity to the wealth and protection of the country."
>
> THOMAS JEFFERSON

hemp harvest for themselves and denying supplies to the British, the colonies stood a better chance of setting themselves up as an independent nation with a self-sufficient economy. Even the first draft of the Declaration of Independence was written on hemp paper.

THE HASHEESH EATER

Hash and marijuana were legal in America and Europe, and the mid-1800s saw a tremendous rise in drug experimentation. Patent medicines containing not only cannabis but opium and other narcotics became very popular amongst the bohemian bourgeoisie; certain artists and intellectuals adopted the practice of eating hashish in underground clubs, and occasionally publishing accounts of their experiences.

One such infamous author was young Fitz Hugh Ludlow, who imbibed a hashish tincture purchased from a New York State apothecary and experimented with its effects on his body and mind, believing that the large doses of hash helped him gain insight into himself and the world. Ludlow published *The Hasheesh Eater* in 1857, at first as an anonymous author; later acclaim turned him into an admired counter-culture figure.

Many influential writers, artists, and intellectuals smoked or ate cannabis in the discreet "hash dens" found in many cities in the late 1800s. Even occultists embraced the exotic intoxicant, using it for sex magic rituals, séances, and to facilitate astral projection. Cannabis became part of a new age menu that included paganism, kundalini yoga, vegetarianism, and other Eastern spiritual ideas like karma and reincarnation. After many hundreds of years in hiding, the witches had emerged again.

> "Ha! What means this sudden thrill? A shock, as of some unimagined vital force, shoots without warning through my entire frame, leaping to my fingers' ends, piercing my brain, startling me till I almost spring from my chair. I could not doubt it. I was in the power of the hasheesh influence."
>
> FITZ HUGH LUDLOW, FROM
> *THE HASHEESH EATER*

ANSLINGER'S REIGN OF TERROR

The unrestrained hedonism of the late 1800s, however, created a backlash.

Starting with the Pure Food and Drug Act in 1906, America's newly powerful pharmaceutical industry sought to eliminate competition from cannabis and other botanical treatments. While medical schools turned away from traditional plant medicine in favor of precisely measured, purified pharmaceutical products, the American Medical Association warned against those who offered traditional folk healing, transforming the practice of modern medicine forever.

Then turn-of-the-century media mogul William Randolph Hearst's newspapers began circulating lurid tales of crimes committed while under the influence of "marihuana" in the 1920s. These stories often linked "dangerous" marijuana use to blacks and Mexicans, whipping up a prurient fear of rape and violence committed by dope-crazed minorities against white folks.

As extensively detailed in former *High Times* editor Larry "Ratso" Sloman's 1979 book *Reefer Madness*, the original campaign by muckraking journalists, power-grabbing politicos, and freaked-out citizens to eradicate marijuana was based on the erroneous idea that cannabis turns ordinary people into desperate addicts driven to maim and murder "just for kicks." Adding to the toxic combination of racism, sensational propaganda, and hysterical fearmongering, Harry J. Anslinger, who was appointed in 1930 as the first head of the Federal Bureau of Narcotics, was determined to illegalize marijuana by any means necessary. Indeed, Anslinger's re-branding of "cannabis" by replacing the scientific name with the Mexican slang term "marihuana" proved successful, since most of the public and many lawmakers failed to realize that these two terms were in fact describing the same plant.

Anslinger set people who'd never used or even seen marijuana against it by compiling a file, used in court testimony, of salacious articles containing the most shocking stories he could find that cast the menace of marijuana as their villain, many from the Hearst newspapers. An often-used favorite of his centered around Victor Licata, a twenty-one-year-old man who murdered his entire family in Tampa, Florida, a horrific crime Anslinger blamed

> *"You smoke a joint and you're likely to kill your brother."*
>
> HARRY J. ANSLINGER, U.S. BUREAU OF NARCOTICS COMMISSIONER 1930–1962

entirely on "the devil's lettuce." The newspaper article mentioned that "the slayer had been smoking marijuana cigarettes for more than six months," but ignored the fact that Licata's criminal insanity was most likely inherited, since his mother and father were first cousins, and his granduncle and several other close relatives had been committed to insane asylums.

A well-coordinated campaign against "marihuana" by Harry J. Anslinger led to Congress passing the Marihuana Tax Act of 1937, which effectively made cannabis illegal by imposing a tax upon its sale or cultivation. Dealers who sold pot without acquiring a tax stamp were arrested, and cannabis became increasingly difficult to obtain. Additional state laws that illegal-

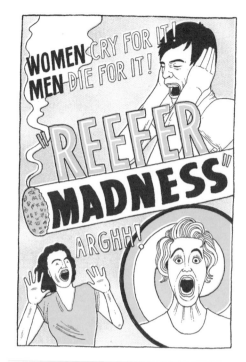

The devil's lettuce.

ized marijuana ended its use as an ingredient in patent medicines. Anslinger then continued his crusade, next targeting musicians (though according to Anslinger, not "good musicians, but the jazz type"). He kept files on many jazz luminaries, including Louis Armstrong, Count Basie, Duke Ellington, and Dizzy Gillespie, and targeted jazz clubs for infiltration by paid informants. The Harlem tea pads—mixed race after-hours parties where blacks and whites socialized openly, sharing reefers and enjoying the music—provoked the most serious enforcement efforts.

A VOICE OF REASON

In 1944, a report commissioned by New York mayor Fiorello La Guardia seriously challenged this anti-reefer hysteria for the first time, by disclosing the findings of a blue-ribbon panel of physicians, psychiatrists, psychologists, pharmacologists, chemists, and sociologists tasked with studying the subject of marijuana. The La Guardia report was the most thorough study of cannabis completed in the United States at that time, and its findings forcefully contradicted Anslinger's well-worn myths. Besides discrediting some obvious misconceptions, such as "The majority of marihuana smokers are Negroes and Latin Americans," and "The distribution and use of marihuana is centered in Harlem," the La Guardia report destroyed several drug war lies that are still used today, confirming most importantly that "The practice of smoking marihuana does not lead to addiction in the medical sense of the word," and "The use of marihuana does not lead to morphine, heroin, or cocaine addiction."

This report from a panel of distinguished scientists and professionals also asserted that marijuana doesn't cause people to commit crimes, is not widely used by schoolchildren, and doesn't lead to juvenile delinquency, ultimately concluding "the publicity concerning the catastrophic effects of marihuana-smoking in New York City is unfounded." Anslinger was enraged at the findings of the La Guardia Committee and declared the report to be "unscientific," and pressured the American Medical Association to prepare a report that would reflect the government's position.

YOU ARE THE ENEMY

Unfortunately, not much changed after the LaGuardia report, because marijuana prohibition had little to do with marijuana, and lots to do with prohibition. Anslinger's lust for power and obsessive focus on demonizing marijuana served the establishment well, by providing a way to assert social control over the undesirable people who used the drug, whether they were Mexican farmhands, Negro jazz musicians, Hollywood actors, communist sympathizers, Beatnik poets, or antiwar protestors.

The demon weed would prove a handy point of law enforcement leverage. After Beat poet and author Allen Ginsberg made several high-profile talk show appearances in the early 1960s to discuss how the marijuana laws were too harsh and make pleas for legalization, the Bureau of Narcotics began investigating him in an attempt to set up a drug bust. According to Sloman, "Marijuana would become a vital armament in a burgeoning counterculture that would spring up in the sixties and manifest itself as a full frontal attack on the social and economic institutions of America. Pot would be politicized, its powers embellished, its myth enlarged, its use further ritualized."

Marijuana increasingly became part of the culture wars, as an aging authoritarian demographic—threatened by these freethinking hippie kids who preached peace and love—used drug laws as a pretext for squashing left-wing groups and subverting their progress. Even after Anslinger's retirement in 1962 at the age of seventy, power-hungry bureaucrats like J. Edgar Hoover targeted civil rights groups, women's rights groups, antiwar groups, the Black Panthers, Students for a Democratic Society, the American Indian Movement, and many others for infiltration and subversion through a secret, illegal program known as COINTELPRO. Often marijuana busts, based on real or "planted" evidence, provided a way to get a foot in the door of these groups, by creating informants or simply jailing the movement and its leaders.

Anslinger's final victory came in 1961, when the United Nations passed the Single Convention on Narcotic Drugs treaty, which made cannabis illegal worldwide and forced participating nations to abide by drug laws adopted by the UN. Post-retirement, Harry was the U.S. Representative to the United Nations Narcotics Commission, and in 1967 he testified before the Senate Foreign Relations Committee arguing for the United States to sign the Single Convention Treaty, proclaiming that this action would allow the United States "to use our treaty obligations to resist legalized use of marijuana." Little media coverage was granted to this momentous decision, and the United States signed onto the treaty in 1968, an agreement which stymies drug reform efforts to this very day.

TRICKY DICK AND THE DAWN OF THE DRUG WAR

When Richard Nixon moved into the White House in 1969, he drew a hard line against the hippies, viewing marijuana "as a useful wedge issue he could play for political advantage," according to Martin A. Lee, author of *Smoke Signals*, an engaging social history of marijuana. Starting with Operation Intercept in 1969, an international drug interdiction effort that tied up traffic at border crossings for miles, Nixon launched his crusade against drug culture, which would ultimately cost taxpayers billions, lock up hundreds of thousands, and block research of cannabis as a life-saving medicine.

In 1970, Congress ratified the Controlled Substances Act, which grouped illicit drugs in different schedules according to their potential for abuse and medical uses. Politicians, not scientists or doctors, marked marijuana as a dangerous drug having no therapeutic value and a high potential for abuse, landing it in the most restrictive Schedule I category alongside heroin.

On June 18, 1971, Nixon held a press conference, declaring drug abuse to be "public enemy number one," and the media popularized the phrase "war on drugs" as a catchall for the United States' new policy of using military intervention and oppressive police tactics to combat the "drug menace."

Continuing the racist underpinnings of the war on drugs, Nixon privately railed against marijuana and "the Jews," remarking to H. R. Haldeman, a close aide, that "every one of those bastards that are out for legalizing marijuana is Jewish. What the Christ is the matter with the Jews?" According to Haldeman's diary,

> "*I now have absolute proof that smoking even one marijuana cigarette is equal in brain damage to being on Bikini Island during an H-bomb blast.*"
>
> RONALD REAGAN

> "Recommendation: Increased support of studies which evaluate the efficacy of Marihuana in the treatment of physical impairments and disease is recommended. Historical references have been noted throughout the literature referring to the use of cannabis products as therapeutically useful agents. Of particular significance for current research with controlled quality, quantity, and therapeutic settings, would be investigations into the treatment of glaucoma, migraine, alcoholism, and terminal cancer. The NIMII-FDA Psychotomimetic Advisory Committee's authorization of studies designed to explore the therapeutic uses of marihuana is commended."
>
> FROM THE 1972 REPORT OF THE NATIONAL COMMISSION ON MARIHUANA AND DRUG ABUSE, *MARIHUANA: A SIGNAL OF MISUNDERSTANDING*

RESCHEDULING *and* DESCHEDULING

❁ ❁ ❁ ❁ ❁ ❁ ❁ ❁ ❁ ❁ ❁

While progress is made toward full legalization, there's a parallel push to try to recategorize marijuana in the DEA's Drug Schedules—five categories under which the government classifies substances and subjects them to levels of enforcement and regulation. Despite substantial evidence to the contrary, marijuana is categorized among the "most dangerous" drugs on the schedule, worse than cocaine and methamphetamine (which are below it in Schedule II).

SCHEDULE I: *Schedule I drugs, substances, or chemicals are defined as drugs with no currently accepted medical use and a high potential for abuse. Schedule I drugs are the most dangerous drugs of all the drug schedules with potentially severe psychological or physical dependence. Some examples of Schedule I drugs are:*

heroin, lysergic acid diethylamide (LSD), marijuana (cannabis), 3,4-methylene-dioxymethamphetamine (ecstasy), methaqualone, and peyote

In early 2014, a group of eighteen federal lawmakers requested that the U.S. Attorney General reclassify marijuana more sensibly, without result. In a statement advocating removing marijuana from the schedule entirely, the group Drug Policy Alliance points to the ineffectiveness of such efforts in the past in a statement:

In 1972, NORML launched the first petition to reschedule marijuana from Schedule I to II. The petition was not given a federal hearing until 1986 and was ultimately denied after over two decades of court challenges— despite the fact that DEA Administrative Law Judge Francis L. Young concluded that marijuana is "one of the safest therapeutically active substances . . . . In strict medical terms, marijuana is far safer than many foods we commonly consume."

In 2002, patient advocates petitioned DEA to move marijuana to Schedule III, IV or V, on the basis of a scientific evaluation. DEA Administrator Michele Leonhart rejected this petition in 2011— after eight years of delay and only after petitioners filed suit.

Even a 2011 petition from a group of sitting governors has gone unanswered.

The group goes on to point out that reducing its classification would not protect state medical marijuana programs, change federal legal penalties, or break the de-facto federal prevention of cannabis research. Descheduling, which could only happen thorough Congressional action, and regulating it similarly to alcohol, is clearly the answer.

the president "emphasized that you have to face that the whole problem is really the blacks. The key is to devise a system that recognizes this while not appearing to." As *Smoke Signals* notes, "the 'system' that Tricky Dick devised in response to this 'problem' was the war on drugs, which would disproportionately target people of color."

Like La Guardia, Nixon commissioned a panel to investigate the marijuana menace, but this time, its members weren't objective professional scientists and doctors, but the president's hand-picked flunkies, anti-drug reactionaries, and lifelong bureaucrats. Still, the Shafer Commission, as this panel was known, released a report in 1972 that wholly validated the arguments made by pro-pot activists. Entitled "Marijuana: A Signal of Misunderstanding," the Shafer Commission report concluded that "Neither the marijuana user or the drug itself can be said to constitute a danger to public safety," recommending

THE NEW JIM CROW

A 2013 report by the American Civil Liberties Union revealed that a person is arrested in the United States every thirty-seven seconds for weed, totaling over eight million pot arrests from 2001 and 2010. These arrests cost taxpayers about 3.6 billion dollars per year, with African Americans almost four times more likely to be popped for pot than whites, despite using marijuana at similar rates.

As director Eugene Jarecki told *High Times* and illustrated in his 2012 anti-drug war documentary *The House I Live In,* "Since Richard Nixon declared the war on drugs in 1971, we have seen a 700 percent increase in our prison population, and about half of those are African Americans."

In her powerful 2010 book *The New Jim Crow,* author Michelle Alexander exposed this system, and urged the civil rights community to reform the laws that warehouse young black men in jails. In a 2013 *New York Times* op-ed, Alexander wrote, "As a parent of black children, I can tell you that I'm far more worried about my kids going to jail and being relegated to a permanent second-class status than getting high."

lifting criminal penalties and funding research into possible medical benefits. Instead, Nixon simply ignored the findings of his own experts and continued the harmful policy of prohibition.

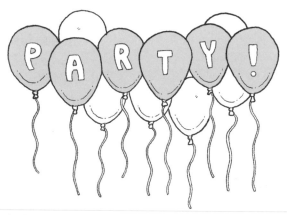

History moves in the right direction.

LEGALIZED IT!

California voters approved America's first state-wide medical marijuana law in 1996, after pioneering marijuana activists like Valerie Corral, Dennis Peron, and "Brownie Mary" Rathbun worked for years to draft and pass California's Prop 215, a truly groundbreaking law protecting patients with a doctor's recommendation to use cannabis from arrest and imprisonment. Each of these compassionate rebels had witnessed firsthand the power of cannabis to soothe seizures, nourish bodies wasting away from AIDS, and strengthen the will of cancer patients who just wanted to survive, and they refused to let the government make the sick and dying casualties of the war on drugs.

In the almost twenty years since the passage of Prop 215, more than twenty other states have joined California in protecting the rights of patients, allowing millions to experience the healing properties of marijuana without legal worry. These patients, in turn, now feel secure enough to speak up to their friends, family, co-workers, and neighbors, forever changing society's attitude toward medical marijuana as a result, simply by relating their positive experiences. In fact, support for medical marijuana nationwide has never been higher, as proven by a Fox News poll released in May 2013, which showed 85 percent of voters believe cannabis use should be legal if authorized by a physician.

The public also increasingly understands that cannabis is far safer to use than pharmaceutical drugs, alcohol, tobacco, and many over-the-counter medications. More than twenty-two thousand people accidentally overdose on prescription drugs each year, while another eighty thousand die from alcohol-related causes—marijuana, in comparison, has no fatal dose. Yet booze and pills remain not just widely available, but enthusiastically promoted during major sporting events and considered an integral part of our culture.

Fed up with watching Americans drink alcohol and smoke cigarettes to unwind from a stressful day or escape their worries, while choosing a far safer alternative lands people in jail, pro-legalization activists decided to fight back by targeting this hypocrisy. Their simple message, "cannabis is safer than alcohol," played a major role in educating the public prior to Election Day 2012, when voters in Colorado and Washington State made history by approving measures legalizing possession of up to an ounce of marijuana for all adults twenty-one and over, plus state-licensed commercial cultivation and sales. Colorado will also allow up to six plants to be grown at home for personal use.

In Washington, endorsements came from prominent law enforcement and public health officials—groups that don't always see eye to eye on drug issues—including Seattle City Attorney Pete Holmes and Mayor Michael McGinn, former U.S. Attorney for the Western District of Washington John McKay (the highest-ranking American law enforcement official ever to support legalization), and State Representative Mary Lou Dickerson. Colorado's Amendment 64 was supported by a broad coalition of city council members, editorial boards from area newspapers, union groups, and local politicians such as U.S. Representative Jared Polis, State Senator Shawn Mitchell, and former U.S. Congressman Tom Tancredo. More than three hundred Colorado physicians endorsed the move to legalize pot, and the

> **"We did not view marijuana as a significant health problem—as it was not. . . . Nobody dies from marijuana. Marijuana smoking, in fact, if one wants to be honest, is a source of pleasure and amusement to countless millions of people in America, and it continues to be that way."**
>
> PETER BOURNE, "DRUG CZAR" DURING THE CARTER ADMINISTRATION

initiative even garnered the support of some unlikely backers, including Pat Robertson, evangelist and founder of the Christian Coalition.

As *High Times* west coast editor David Bienenstock noted in his triumphant 2013 article "Legalized It!,"

Neither state's governor supported passage of the initiatives, but both have vowed to faithfully implement the new laws. Though Colorado's John Hickenlooper—who made his fortune as proprietor of Denver's first brew pub—apparently couldn't help but greet his constituents' clear desire for a safer legal alternative to alcohol with a lame pot joke at their expense.

"The voters have spoken, and we have to respect their will," he commented on election night, after Amendment 64 legalized marijuana with 55 percent in favor. "This will be a complicated process, but we intend to follow through. That said, federal law still says marijuana is an illegal drug, so don't break out the Cheetos or Goldfish too quickly."

With legalization in Colorado and Washington State sparking debate about drug law reform around the world, activists remain cautiously optimistic about the federal government's reaction. As Bienenstock notes, "For now, the U.S. Department of Justice has decided to let both Colorado and Washington go forward with implementing legal marijuana, so long as their regulatory systems maintain tight control over cultivation and sales. . . ." An August 2013 directive from Attorney General Eric Holder outlined the federal government's permissive attitude toward the legalization experiments proceeding out west, while reserving the federal

> **"The amount of money and of legal energy being given to prosecute hundreds of thousands of Americans who are caught with a few ounces of marijuana in their jeans simply makes no sense—the kindest way to put it. A sterner way to put it is that it is an outrage, an imposition on basic civil liberties and on the reasonable expenditure of social energy."**
>
> WILLIAM F. BUCKLEY

government's right to prosecute people for distributing marijuana to minors, providing cash to cartels, bringing pot over state lines, driving under the influence, and growing cannabis on public land, among other violations of new state laws.

GREEN WEDNESDAY

On New Year's Day 2014, jubilant crowds gathered in Colorado to experience opening day for the state's new retail pot stores, waiting in lines for hours to be treated like customers rather than criminals. Twenty-four marijuana shops opened on "Green Wednesday," as the historic occasion came to be known, with media outlets reporting "over one million dollars in sales in a single day." At a press conference held that morning by Amendment 64 proponents, co-director Mason Tvert stated, "Millions of adults use marijuana in the United States. Only in Colorado will they be purchasing it from legitimate, regulated businesses instead of in the underground market. It won't be long before other states follow suit."

420 FRIENDLY

Today, 4/20 has gone mainstream as the homegrown holiday grows in popularity every year, but it started out as a very humble smoking ceremony. During a 2006 interview, *High Times* editor Steve Hager explained the origins of 4/20 to ABC News. Hager's investigation into the origins of 420 as a cannabis code revealed that the trend began with a group of San Rafael high school students in 1971. Dubbed "the Waldos," this crew would meet at 4:20 to smoke weed, and over time the number was adopted as a code for getting high. The message of 420 spread through the Grateful Dead subculture in Marin County before being publicized by *High Times* in 1991, leading stoners worldwide to adopt it as shorthand for "cannabis smoking," to be celebrated every day at 4:20 P.M. and all day on April 20, which has become the "Thanksgiving of smoking pot!"

CANADIAN CANNABIS

Along with Israel and the Netherlands, Canada is one of the few nations with a comprehensive medical marijuana program. Starting in April 2014, Canada is poised to shift its system from a citizen-based cultivation program with patients and designated caregivers growing medicine to a privatized and tightly regulated plan in which "a handful of corporations will now be exclusively authorized to grow medical pot in Canada," says *High Times* Canadian correspondent Eric Biksa. The new system will require patients to complete an application, submit a doctor's note, and wait for corporate approval. Once authorized, patients will place orders for cannabis and have it delivered to their door via a secure courier service. Canada expects up to 450,000 people to take advantage of this program by 2024, and Biksa remarks, "However the new system pans out, one thing is clear: Large-scale production that can deliver both consistent and reliable high-quality results is the new challenge that must be met."

Since that historic day, the tremendous tax windfall of legal pot has certainly raised eyebrows in other states that are now considering following suit. Colorado Governor John Hickenlooper's budget office "expects the recreational and medical marijuana industries will pump nearly $134 million in tax and fee revenue into state coffers in the fiscal year beginning in July 2014," according to the *Denver Post*, exceeding previous estimates by more than 50 percent. The Associated Press reported that legal marijuana in Washington State will "bring nearly $190 million to state coffers over a four-year period starting in mid-2015," according to a prediction from the Economic and Revenue Forecast Council.

Inspired by this rapidly shifting political landscape in the United States, leaders throughout Latin America have increasingly called for a debate on drug law reform.

In Uruguay, President José Mujica has decided not to wait for any further analysis. In December 2013, he signed a legalization bill that will allow any citizen over eighteen years of age to cultivate personal amounts of cannabis, while pharmacies will sell the herb over the counter to residents. By making Uruguay the first country to legalize cannabis production and sales, President Mujica intends to wrestle the trade away from organized crime syndicates, remarking to NBC News that "we've given this market as a gift to the drug traffickers and that is more destructive socially than the drug itself, because it rots the whole of society."

Battered by a global drug war that costs exorbitant sums of money and ruins countless lives, leaders around the world have been watching progress in Uruguay and planning reforms of their own. In 2016, the United Nation' General Assembly will hold a special session on the prohibition of drugs, providing the global community an opportunity to amend the Single Convention Treaty to allow for cannabis and hemp production.

In a revealing January 2014 interview with *The New Yorker*, President Obama opened up about his feelings on pot use, saying "I don't think it is more dangerous than alcohol," echoing the main talking point that pro-pot activists hammered home in Colorado. Obama went on to decry the racial disparities in drug sentencing, before asserting that "we should not be locking up kids or individual users for long stretches of jail time when some of the folks who are writing those laws have probably done the same thing."

Dr. Lester Grinspoon, associate professor emeritus at Harvard Medical School and author of *Marihuana Reconsidered* (1971) writes frequently about medical marijuana, and is something of an elder statesman when

> **"Middle-class kids don't get locked up for smoking pot, and poor kids do. . . . And African American kids and Latino kids are more likely to be poor and less likely to have the resources and the support to avoid unduly harsh penalties. . . . We should not be locking up kids or individual users for long stretches of jail time when some of the folks who are writing those laws have probably done the same thing."**
>
> BARACK OBAMA

KNOW YOUR RIGHTS

Marijuana isn't fully legal in most places (yet), so be sure to remember that fact and be safe. If you are encountered by law enforcement, remember to stay calm, cool, and use these commonsense tips from the National Organization to Reform Marijuana Laws (norml.org) to avoid getting in trouble.

Don't leave contraband in plain view. If a cop at your front door can look through the window and see you hitting a bong, then they can easily go get a warrant to come in. Be sure to keep your stash and any and all paraphernalia put away in drawers or cabinets. This is also important in your car—don't leave roaches in the ashtray!

Do not consent. Never consent to a search. Politely but firmly refuse to be searched, and say "I do not consent to a search of my [person, baggage, purse, luggage, vehicle, house, blood, etc.] I do not consent to this contact and do not want to answer any questions. If I am not under arrest, I would like to go now (or be left alone)."

Don't answer questions without an attorney present. Anything you say to anyone can be used against you. You have the right to have an attorney present during questioning and you should use it. If you are arrested, do not answer any questions and get an attorney as soon as possible.

Determine if you can leave. Unless you are being detained under police custody or arrested, then you can stop contact with law enforcement. You can ask officers, "Am I under arrest or otherwise detained?" If the answer is, "No," you may leave. When an officer attempts to contact or question you, you should politely say: "I do not consent to this contact and I do not want to answer any questions. If I am not under arrest I would like to go now (or be left alone)."

Do not be hostile and do not physically resist. Sometimes cops do not follow protocol and will detain, search, and arrest those who have not consented. It's important not to resist, never consent, stay polite, and get an attorney immediately.

 Learn more and download a "Freedom Card" to carry in your wallet at norml.org.

A SHORT HISTORY OF
HIGH TIMES

In 1974, the first issue of *High Times* hit the newsstands, published by an outlaw pot smuggler known as Tom Forçade. His real name was Gary Goodson, but back when he was a teenager in Arizona, everyone called him "Junior." Junior Goodson was a hotrod hell-raiser who would regularly outrace the Utah State Highway Patrol just for fun in car chases on the Bonneville Salt Flats. Junior eventually turned his adolescent preoccupation with fast cars and adrenalized adventure into a successful career as a first-class marijuana smuggler. He changed his name and quickly moved on to boats and planes as his favored mode of illicit expression.

"There are only two kinds of pot dealers," Forçade used to say: "those who need a fork lift and those who don't. And I'm the kind who needs a fork lift."

Tom was much more than an uncommonly good drug smuggler, however: He was a writer, an editor, a publisher, and a movie producer. He founded the Underground Press Syndicate, which linked, in content and style, many of the ad hoc countercultural magazines and newspapers that had popped up around the country.

Tom Forçade's *High Times* was marked by vibrant concept covers that harked back to the bygone days of the great periodicals. It was a fat magazine noted for its in-depth stories on exotic drugs penned by savvy writers, and for paraphernalia ads that seemed to come from another world. Tom's *High Times* was the first periodical to publish four-color photos of desiccated flowers pressed into brick and call this beauty . . . and so the "bud shot" was born.

Further traditions emerged when Bob Marley became the first celebrity to pose for a *High Times* cover with an unwise quantity of weed, and when Trans High Market Quotations (THMQ) allowed stoners their first view of the street price of marijuana. Beginning with the second issue, Tom also gave a full page of advertising every month to the National Organization for the Reform of Marijuana Laws (NORML). At his behest, *High Times* became NORML's largest corporate donor as well, a tradition that has continued unbroken to this day.

—Richard Cusik

it comes to advocacy for legalizing marijuana. He had this optimistic reaction to his home state of Massachusetts approving medical marijuana in the same election as the Colorado and Washington wins: "For me, it was a truly historic night, because the end of alcohol prohibition started with the states, and I believe the same thing will happen with marijuana."

At the time of this writing, cheered by these recent events, many activists feel the walls of pot prohibition have begun to tumble down, and that we've truly reached a "spliffing point" where real change is within reach. The year this book is published will also mark the fortieth anniversary of *High Times* magazine, and so we, too, are looking forward to the bright green future of fully legal pot with incredible optimism and anticipation.

May the future lead to even Higher Times!

The Science of Cannabis

PROOF AND POTENTIAL

If time-traveling marijuana enthusiasts from the year 2050 appeared in the here and now and claimed that the adoption of cannabis-based medicines was heralded in their future society as a scientific advancement on par with penicillin or the polio vaccine, plenty of people would believe them. Despite the longstanding chokehold of government restrictions on marijuana research, what objective studies we do have point to its potential medical benefits, and with the advent of medical-marijuana laws in 1996, the anecdotal evidence of the herb's many healing properties just keeps piling up, along with serious, peer-reviewed research and revolutionary studies into the anti-cancer and pro-health attributes of this ancient botanical medicine.

In fact, were this plant just now discovered deep in the Amazon, or reintroduced to society under any other name but the much-maligned "marijuana," the mainstream media would breathlessly proclaim it as a miracle "neutraceutical" like acai, yacon, or spirulina—only so much more! For what other plant known to man is effective against epilepsy, cancer, Alzheimer's, Crohn's, multiple sclerosis, and arthritis while providing a pleasant mental diversion and stress relief?

Until substantial changes in the law allow scientists and doctors to freely study marijuana's full potential, we still have a lot to learn. But let's start with what we already know, including the overwhelming evidence that cannabis is a safe, effective medicine in its natural form.

HOW DOES GETTING HIGH WORK?

First, you ingest the dried, cured flowers of cannabis or its concentrated resin, known as hash, most commonly by smoking, vaporizing, or eating it. Fresh cannabis isn't psychoactive at all, and the plant must be dried or heated to convert acidic cannabinoids like THCA into psychedelic THC.

When this happens—for sake of example, let's say you've just smoked it—marijuana's active chemical components, including THC and other cannabinoids, are absorbed by the alveoli in your lungs and pass into your bloodstream, where they move quickly to your brain. The fast-acting "high" that results from smoking happens when that THC binds to specific cannabinoid receptors throughout your brain and body. As seasoned pot smokers know, this process can take place in mere minutes, which makes controlling your dose easy when ingesting through the lungs by smoking or vaporizing. Because the effects come on so rapidly, you can stop when you've had enough and then easily adjust with a puff or two later if necessary. The high continues for about an hour or so before it wears off entirely, though THC can remain detectable in your body for as long as ten days to a month after inhalation. This is why marijuana is the most commonly found substance in drug testing (see p. 48).

Vaporization works by boiling beneficial cannabinoids found in resinous balls on the plant until they release as a fine vapor, which happens at a temperature below the point of combustion. The technique has been practiced in some form since the sixties, but modern technology has lately made it a lot more convenient, efficient, and cost effective, leading to a surge of interest. Vaporization also avoids the harmful byproducts of combustion, which can lead to respiratory irritation.

Eating cannabis gets you high in a different, more intense way because your liver converts THC into a chemical called 11-hydroxy THC that's far stronger than the THC that's absorbed through your lungs. The process of digestion

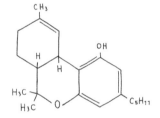

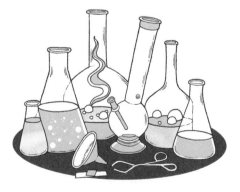

The THC molecule. Research continues to reveal more about the effects and benefits of cannabis.

and absorption into your bloodstream can take up to two hours or more when eating, depending on what you've consumed that day, your weight, and your metabolism. This can all contribute to getting higher than you want to when the full effects kick in (especially if you've impatiently scarfed another magic brownie). For advice for consuming edibles, see p. 125.

Most users of cannabis report feelings of bliss, relaxation, and enhancement of sensual stimuli. Appetite is increased, libido is invigorated, pain is relieved, laughter is encouraged, and creative ideas are generated after inhaling or ingesting cannabis. Common side effects of cannabis smoking include red eyes and cottonmouth. Weed decreases ocular pressure and increases blood flow, so your eyes get bloodshot for the same reason cannabinoids work for treating glaucoma. Cottonmouth happens because cannabinoids interact with

WHAT'S A CANNABINOID?

🍁 🍁 🍁 🍁 🍁 🍁 🍁 🍁 🍁 🍁

🍁 **Cannabinoid:** Chemical compounds which act on cannabinoid receptors in cells found throughout the human body.

🍁 **Endocannabinoid:** Cannabinoid produced in the bodies of mammals, including humans.

🍁 **Phytocannabinoids:** Cannabinoid produced in the cannabis plant. There are eighty-five different known phytocannabinoids.

🍁 **Cannabinoid receptors:** A type of cell membrane receptor involved in a variety of physiological processes, including appetite, pain-sensation, mood, and memory.

🍁 **THC:** Delta-9-tetrahydrocannabinol, the main psychoactive cannabinoid found in the cannabis plant.

🍁 **CBD:** Cannabidiol, a cannabinoid which confounds THC and lessens psychoactivity. Also relieves convulsions, nausea, inflammation, and anxiety.

receptors at the saliva glands, so be sure to drink plenty of water during a smoke session to avoid any annoying dryness.

CANNABIS CHEMISTRY

Most pot enthusiasts have heard of THC ("It's the chemical in pot that makes you high!"), but few have ever really delved into the complex and fascinating world of cannabis chemistry, where new discoveries continue to reveal the powerful healing properties of this amazing natural medicine.

Pioneering research on these properties began in Israel in 1964, when a scientist named Dr. Raphael Mechoulam first isolated the plant's primary psychoactive constituent, Delta 9-tetrahydrocannabinol, also known as THC.

Mechoulam's groundbreaking research also eventually led to the discovery of dozens of other active chemical compounds in cannabis, known as cannabinoids, including cannabidiol (CBD); the discovery of cannabinoid receptors in the human brain; and, notably, the endocannabinoid system in the human body that the cannabis compounds interact with. It's important to note that there are *endo*cannabinoids, which are produced inside human beings, and *phyto*cannabinoids, which are found only in the cannabis plant. We now know that ingesting marijuana affects your body via receptors (called CB1 and CB2) found in the brain and throughout the human organism that function only when engaged by a cannabinoid.

Only a few of cannabis's eighty-five known cannabinoids can attach to these receptors, including THC, THCV, CBG, and other cannabinoids just now being studied. CBD does not connect with either CB1 or CB2, but does interact with the body in other ways to produce relief from anxiety, inflammation, nausea, and convulsions.

YOUR INNER CANNABINOIDS

Receptors like CB1 and CB2 exist as part of the endogenous cannabinoid system, which regulates appetite, sensitivity to pain, mood, emotions, and aspects of memory. The body has these receptors all over it, which explains how cannabis can be so helpful for such a wide variety of medical conditions. The compound in the human brain that activates these receptors is known as *anandamide*, a neurotransmitter named for the Sanskrit word *ananda*, which means "bliss" or "delight."

IS SMOKING POT *BAD* FOR ME?

🌿 🌿 🌿 🌿 🌿 🌿 🌿 🌿 🌿 🌿

The health risks and benefits of smoking remain controversial, partially because even though it's been proven that pot smokers are less likely to develop lung cancer than tobacco smokers (or even non-smokers), "burning one down" still releases toxic by-products like polycyclic aromatic hydrocarbons, benzopyrene, and carbon monoxide. Cannabis smoke does possess protective anti-cancer properties, as proven by the landmark 2006 Tashkin study conducted at University of California at Los Angeles, that balance out its carcinogens, but smokers should still be aware that long-term heavy use increases the risk of contracting chronic obstructive pulmonary disorder (COPD) and bronchial infections.

Meanwhile, a study conducted by the University of California at San Francisco and the University of Alabama at Birmingham, published in the January 2012 issue of the *Journal of the American Medical Association*, substantiated the fact that a moderate amount of pot smoke doesn't damage the lungs.

Conducted over a period of twenty years, that long-term comprehensive study of 5,115 young adults found that pot smoking was as common as cigarette smoking among the participants. Turns out, lung function among the tobacco smokers predictably decreased over time, while low to moderate pot users actually showed increased lung capacity compared to nonsmokers on two different tests: the total volume of air exhaled and the amount of air exhaled in the first second, both measured following the subject's deepest breath.

Even for prolific pot smokers, the results were the same as nonsmokers, and there was no decline in lung capacity for total air volume exhaled even with the heaviest of tokers. When it came to interpreting the results, some researchers hypothesized that the chemical properties of cannabis protect and possibly even strengthen the lungs.

Professor Robert Melamede, Ph.D. in molecular biology and biochemistry and an expert on the endocannabinoid system, described it to *High Times* in this way: "All people make marijuana-like compounds known as endocannabinoids. Whenever anyone gets hungry, they are giving themselves the 'munchies' with the cannabinoids that they produce. In fact, cannabinoids control every system in the human body (cardiovascular, nervous, endocrine, immune, digestive, reproductive, excretory, musculo-sketetal). It is because of their all-pervasive activity that cannabinoids have an impact on so many illnesses.

"Cannabinoids kill many types of cancer cells, protect against Alzheimer's disease, delay the onset and severity of auto-immune diseases such as arthritis, diabetes, multiple sclerosis, and Crohn's disease, and recently have been shown to both protect the heart from damage as well as to protect against arteriosclerosis. They relieve pain, stimulate the appetite, and promote sound sleep. Cannabinoids also regulate stress, learning, and open-mindedness."

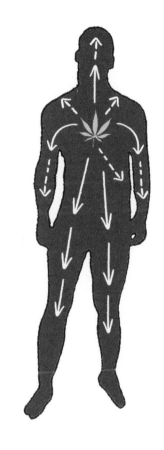

The endocannabinoid system interacts with many other systems in the body.

Dr. Melamede and other scientists have advanced a theory that phytocannabinoids can be essential supplements that help keep human beings healthy. Which begs the question: If endocannabinoids modulate many of the body's systems, would naturally low levels make a person more susceptible to illness?

Dr. Ethan Russo thinks so, calling the syndrome an endogenous cannabinoid deficiency disorder in his research papers, and theorizing it could be responsible for the underlying cause of many illnesses. A senior medical adviser to the Cannabinoid Research Institute established by GW Pharmaceuticals, Dr. Russo considers it possible that some people don't manufacture enough cannabinoids on their own, and this can lead to irritable bowel syndrome, glaucoma, and migraines, as well as many other, far more serious problems.

While more research is required and no single case contains all the answers, the remarkable story of a California medical marijuana patient named Kristen Peskuski illustrates a possible case of endocannabinoid deficiency. For her entire life, Kristen suffered from various ailments including lupus, rheumatoid arthritis, endometriosis, interstitial cystitis, hypoglycemia, anemia, chronic sinusitis, and chronic bacterial infections. After discovering that smoking a little weed really helped her various conditions, Kristen began to do research into the endocannabinoid system, and what she discovered changed her life.

As documented by Kym Kemp for *High Times Medical Marijuana* magazine in her 2010 article "Raw Medicine," Kristen left her home in the Midwest and moved to California in order to saturate her body with cannabinoids. Kemp writes, "All along, Kristen's doctors had studied different parts of her body and treated different things that went wrong with them, but they hadn't been looking at the whole picture. The root of her problems, she came to believe, was that she needed to replace the cannabinoids her body failed to produce naturally."

After meeting Dr. William Courtney, a practitioner of cannabis medicine in Mendocino County, Peskuski began juicing raw cannabis leaves, fresh off the plant, a method of medicating that delivers high levels of healing cannabinoids without any psychoactivity at all. This is because the raw plant only contains acidic cannabinoids, and some form of heating or drying must take place to convert the non-psychoactive acidic form of THC (called THCA) into the psychedelic form we all know and love. Absorbing "straight" acidic cannabinoids in their fresh form allows a patient to receive a much larger amount of healing medicine without being limited by a debilitating high.

After a few years of a solid cannabinoid saturation regimen, Kristen regained her health completely and was even able to carry a successful pregnancy to term after countless doctors in her past had warned that due to her endometriosis, she would never be able to have children.

Kristen's incredible story is just one of many. In fact, a whole new culture of "medical refugees" has been created as those in serious need uproot themselves and then transplant to states where laws protect medical marijuana use. For hundreds of thousands of patients, access to cannabinoids is the difference between life and death.

BLOCKING THE RECEPTORS

If properly functioning and fully engaged cannabinoid receptors are so vital to the proper functioning of the human body, what would happen if you blocked them completely?

In 2007, a weight-loss drug called Rimonabant, produced by pharmaceutical giant Sanofi-Aventis, was withdrawn from the market after reports surfaced of severe depression and even suicides resulting from its use. Marketed under the brand name Acomplia, the drug blocked CB1 receptors, with the intended purpose of helping overweight people melt inches off their waistlines by reducing overall appetite—basically, stopping the body's natural "munchies" before they start. It had the notable side effect that anybody on the drug who smoked, ate, or otherwise ingested pot would find themselves completely unable to get high, since the drug prevents THC or any other cannabinoids from binding to the receptor sites.

The good news is that blocking CB1 did help some people lose weight. But Acomplia also affected emotions and mood so drastically that it was finally deemed too dangerous to ingest. What we learn from the terrible debacle of this anti-obesity drug is that a malfunctioning endocannabinoid system leads to serious negative consequences. And the complex and profound way in which cannabis and its components interact with the body should not be underestimated.

THE POT PILL

The modern desire to isolate components of plants and refine them into pure drugs, coupled with the federal government's need for some response to a growing medical marijuana movement, led the pharmaceutical companies to introduce Marinol, a synthetic THC pill, in 1985.

As researcher Fred Garner notes in the pages of *High Times Medical Marijuana*, "When the U.S. Food and Drug Administration first approved Marinol (pure, synthetic THC), the public was told that a pill containing the active ingredient in marijuana, precisely dosed, was now available by prescription. Experienced marijuana users who tried Marinol disputed this claim: They reported that Marinol produced heavier, more sedating effects and insisted that something in the herb besides delta-9-THC must be biologically active. The so-called 'pot pill,' many suspected, was a ploy to uphold the government's prohibition of the plant itself."

Gardner goes on to explain that cannabis as a natural medicine functions differently than refined, isolated pharmaceutical drugs. Indeed, Dr. Ethan Russo's "entourage effect" research has established a basic working theory that the medical efficacy of cannabis is much greater than the sum of its parts: meaning all of the cannabinoids, terpenes, and flavonoids naturally found in the plant work together in a synergistic fashion to fight disease and promote wellness.

Terpenes, or terpenoids, which we'll discuss more later (see "Aroma Therapy," p. 47), are the chemicals that give cannabis its flavor and aroma, while flavonoids give cannabis flowers and leaves their varying colors of green, gold, purple, red, and orange. On their own, cannabinoids like THC and CBD are odorless and flavorless.

IN SEARCH OF CBD

Though far less well known or understood than its highly psychoactive cousin THC, cannabidiol (CBD) increasingly shows promise in treating pain, insomnia, nausea, anxiety, spasticity, MS, Alzheimer's, and cancer. Researchers have theorized that CBD strongly supports the work of the body's natural immune system, acting as a powerful anti-inflammatory while providing therapeutic benefits to those suffering from a wide range of ailments without any of the (sometimes) unpleasant side effects associated with ingesting high levels of THC.

DR. SANJAY GUPTA: WHY I CHANGED MY MIND ON WEED

🌿 🌿 🌿 🌿 🌿 🌿 🌿 🌿 🌿 🌿

Indicative of the quickly shifting opinion about marijuana in the mainstream and medical communities, CNN's chief medical correspondent and one of America's best-known doctors, neurosurgeon Dr. Sanjay Gupta, published an August 2013 op-ed entitled "Why I Changed My Mind on Weed," writing:

> I traveled around the world to interview medical leaders, experts, growers, and patients. I spoke candidly to them, asking tough questions. What I found was stunning.

> Long before I began this project, I had steadily reviewed the scientific literature on medical marijuana from the United States and thought it was fairly unimpressive. Reading these papers five years ago, it was hard to make a case for medicinal marijuana. I even wrote about this in a TIME magazine article, back in 2009, titled "Why I Would Vote No on Pot."

> Well, I am here to apologize.

> I apologize because I didn't look hard enough, until now. I didn't look far enough. I didn't review papers from smaller labs in other countries doing some remarkable research, and I was too dismissive of the loud chorus of legitimate patients whose symptoms improved on cannabis.

Taking issue with the U.S. Drug Enforcement Agency's placing marijuana in its category of most dangerous drugs, with (according to the Justice Department) "no currently accepted medical use and a high potential for abuse," Gupta states plainly: "We have been terribly and systematically misled for nearly seventy years in the United States."

> They didn't have the science to support that claim, and I now know that when it comes to marijuana neither of those things are true. It doesn't have a high potential for abuse, and there are very legitimate medical applications. In fact, sometimes marijuana is the only thing that works. . . . It is irresponsible not to provide the best care we can as a medical community, care that could involve marijuana.

In March 2014, he updated his position after having met with "hundreds of patients, dozens of scientists and the curious majority who simply want a deeper understanding of this ancient plant."

> I am more convinced than ever that it is irresponsible to not provide the best care we can, care that often may involve marijuana.

> I am not backing down on medical marijuana; I am doubling down.

Because CBD isn't very psychoactive—in fact, it confounds THC by activating cytochrome P450, an enzyme that metabolizes THC—and most users want to get as high as possible, breeders over the years naturally selecting for plants with the highest levels of THC have inadvertently bred a lot of CBD out of the cannabis gene pool. This effectively relegated CBD to the ashtray of history's overlooked cannabinoids until recently, when the surging demand for lab-tested medicine lead to the rediscovery of CBD and increased appreciation of its incredible healing properties.

CBD balances psychoactivity, removing some of the paranoid, edgy, agitated feelings that can result from an overload of too much THC, and providing a nice, relaxing effect. So high-CBD strains are much appreciated by cannabis-naive patients and those who want to provide marijuana medicine to terminally ill children without getting them too high.

Again, more research is needed. But it appears that plants with a THC to CBD ratio of around 1:1 provide the maximum amount of healing. A Spanish seed company called Reggae Seeds has even begun breeding strains with this 1:1 ratio, such as Juanita La Lagrimosa and Dancehall, a two-time winner in European cannabis competitions.

High Times west coast editor David Bienenstock's article "In Search of CBD" explored how the development of a large medical marijuana analytic lab testing industry helped shed light on the problem of CBD depletion. "As the medical marijuana industry established itself in California, Colorado, and elsewhere, an increasing number of collectives and dispensaries started having their medicine lab tested for potency before offering it to patients. And when it came to CBD, the news wasn't good—for while the top dispensaries' medical marijuana consistently tested at 15 percent or higher for THC, very few of those same samples came close to even one percent for CBD.

"Worried by these results, Project CBD—a collaborative effort among physicians, researchers, cannabis-testing laboratories, and medical-marijuana patients and providers—began a pilot program in 2008 that had Oakland's Steep Hill Lab test tens of thousands of samples provided by Harborside Health Center, the single largest cannabis dispensary in the nation, for potency. To their dismay, they discovered that only one in every 750 examples could be defined as 'CBD-rich' (using 4 percent of dried weight as the cutoff), while an even more minuscule percentage reached 8 percent CBD or higher."

As more people became aware of the potential cancer-fighting and pain-relieving properties of CBD, more research is being done to identify and preserve important strains designated as CBD-rich and popularize them among cultivators. High-CBD strains in circulation today include Harlequin, Sour Tsunami, and AC/DC.

In addition to THC and CBD, researchers have now begun to look at cannabinoids that may have medical benefits, including cannabinol (CBN), cannabigerol (CBG), and tetrahydrocannabivarin (THCV or THV).

AROMA THERAPY

Terpenes (or terpenoids) are the chemical components of cannabis responsible for its enticing aroma. They also work in tandem with cannabinoids to provide specific, quantifiable medical benefits.

While phytocannabinoids exist naturally only in the cannabis plant, terpenes are found in many different plant species, including limonene (lemons), myrcene (mangoes), alpha-pinene (pine trees), linalool (coriander), beta-caryophyllene (cloves), and nerolidol (ginger). When it comes to cannabis, these volatile oils evaporate readily, so growers must carefully process, dry, and store their buds to get the most out of their terpenes: and not just their heady bouquet, but also some serious healing properties.

Limonene, found in lemons as well as your bag of Super Lemon Haze, has been found to reduce depression in hospital patients exposed to its fragrance. Pot that smells like pine contains alpha-pinene, known to be a broncodilator with antibacterial and antibiotic properties. Myrcene, a terpenoid found in all mangoes and some marijuana, is anti-inflammatory and sedative. And so on.

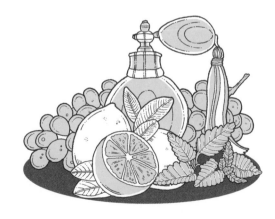

Terpenes are responsible for cannabis' enticing aroma.

LAB TESTED, PATIENT APPROVED

Over the last five years, the rapid rise of analytic laboratories specializing in testing cannabis potency and purity in states with legal medical marijuana has had a profound effect on everyone who grows or uses pot, no matter where they live. For starters, after years of best guessing and heatedly debating which strains had the most THC, we can finally access real, scientific data. Proper testing also ensures a supply of marijuana that's free of mold, pests, chemical residue, and other possible contaminants.

Labs have sprung up nationwide to provide this service, including in Colorado and Washington, the first two fully legal states, which have both mandated that all cannabis sold in retail stores must be tested first.

Determining a desirable dosage through lab testing has also been essential to the rapid growth of the cannabis-infused edibles industry. Since cannabis-laced foods are so powerful, it's vitally important not to eat too much. But before lab testing, there was really no way to know how much

DRUG TESTS

Even in this wonderful new era of legal weed, far too many Americans will face a urine test in the next year. Aside from being an incredible invasion of privacy, drug tests can also detect marijuana in your system for up to a month, meaning cannabis users are often penalized for smoking pot responsibly at home because such tests fail to show impairment, only use. The tests are also, according to the National Workrights Institute, highly dubious. After an extensive study, in fact, the group concluded that "certified drug testing laboratories have significant reliability problems and that the government's assurances that false positive test results are a thing of the past is untrue."

THC was present in an old hippie's homemade brownies or a Phish Head's parking lot goo balls—you just bought the ticket and took the ride, as Hunter S. Thompson used to say.

Now, professionally packaged candy bars with precisely dosed segments containing 45 milligrams of THC each can be obtained in every medical marijuana state. This is a serious boon for everyone who wants to enjoy the relaxing effects of edibles without sleeping for fourteen hours or experiencing a panic attack from an overdose of THC.

CANNABIS VS. CANCER

About ten years ago, cannabis patients, researchers, and doctors started talking openly about the potential for cannabis to treat and possibly even cure certain types of cancer. It remains a controversial subject, but the evidence to support this assertion is compelling, and continues to mount.

Most people already know that marijuana can work wonders for those dealing with the debilitating side effects of chemotherapy, which include nausea, pain, and loss of appetite. Surviving such treatments is actually a great stride toward beating the disease, and so it's a huge benefit that cancer patients are able to deal with chemo treatments far better when medicating with marijuana. But even as early as 1975, researchers had a clue that something bigger than symptom relief might be going on.

That year, the *Journal of the National Cancer Institute* published a paper titled "Anti-cancer Activity of Cannabinoids," by a team of researchers from the Virginia Commonwealth University. Many in the scientific community laughed it off as a fluke due to the cultural climate of drug war, even though the results were quite compelling, including the finding that THC "demonstrated a dose-dependent action of retarded tumor growth," meaning that orally-administered cannabinoids given to mice slowed the growth of their tumors.

> "The illegality of cannabis is outrageous, an impediment to full utilization of a drug which helps produce the serenity and insight, sensitivity, and fellowship so desperately needed in this increasingly mad and dangerous world."
>
> CARL SAGAN

Instead of following up on these promising results, however, the research was abandoned due to political interference during the early days of Nixon's war on drugs.

In fact, the study is one of many cited by the National Cancer Institute, who maintains a list of research with findings of potential benefits, including:

- cannabinoids appear to kill tumor cells

- CBD induces programmed cell death in breast cancer cell lines

- phyto- and endocannabinoids could reduce the risk of colorectal cancer

- cannabinoids modulate pain by reducing inflammation

WHY IS RESEARCH SO DIFFICULT?

In short: the federal government. Brad Burge is director of communications of Multidisciplinary Association for the Study of Psychedelics (MAPS), which pushes the DEA, the National Institute on Drug Abuse (NIDA) and other government agencies to make marijuana research available for studies into its benefits. In his 2010 *High Times Medical Marijuana* article, "Experimenting with Marijuana," he lays out the problem as it frustratingly still persists today. "Since 1968, the federal government has maintained a monopoly on the supply of marijuana for research. Currently, the University of Mississippi houses the only DEA-licensed production facility in the country, under the ownership of Dr. Mahmoud ElSohly, who has an exclusive contract with the NIDA. This means that even if the FDA approves a study, NIDA can still decide not to sell marijuana to the researchers, making the study impossible to conduct. NIDA has already denied marijuana to two MAPS–sponsored, FDA–approved studies."

It's a catch-22: The Feds continue to claim that there's no evidence marijuana in its natural form has medical value while blocking the necessary research from taking place. But when the National Cancer Institute (a part of the NIH) lists the anti-cancer effects of cannabis on its own website, the official federal denials

> "Why is marijuana against the law? It grows naturally upon our planet. Doesn't the idea of making nature against the law seem to you a bit … unnatural?"
>
> BILL HICKS

HIGH MAINTENANCE: FINDING THE *RIGHT* DISPENSARY

☘ ☘ ☘ ☘ ☘ ☘ ☘ ☘ ☘ ☘ ☘

When dispensaries first appeared in otherwise vacant storefronts, strip malls, and office space, the ambiance of such establishments was sometimes little more than "two stoned guys playing video games." Over time, these revolutionary retailers added more services and features, such as alternative health treatments, support groups, social networking, and political activism. Look for dispensaries headed by prominent cannabis activists, since these places will offer a better vibe than purely profit-driven, fly-by-night operations. Seek out dispensaries that stock high quality, lab-tested strains plus a wide variety of edibles and topicals—places that give back to their communities and strive to become cultural centers deserve your support, too. Today, finding the dispensary that's right for you is easier than ever with a search of the online reviews. Web giant Weedmaps.com searches for locations near you, plus provides menus and reviews, along with Leafly.com and good ol' Yelp!

seem like outright hypocrisy. Consistent with NIDA's mission to prove that marijuana is a "bad drug" of abuse (its stated aim is to wipe out all marijuana use), they blatantly refuse to provide cannabis to studies that intend to find evidence of beneficial medicinal properties. It's harder still then to square this stance with the government's securing for itself Patent 6630507, in 2003, covering "Cannabinoids as Antioxidants and Neuroprotectants." In making their case for the patent, the Federal Department of Health and Human Services stated unequivocally that "cannabinoids are found to have particular application as neuroprotectants, for example in limiting neurological damage following lack of blood-flow to the brain, such as stroke and trauma, or in the treatment of neurodegenerative diseases, such as Alzheimer's disease, Parkinson's disease, and HIV dementia."

Fortunately, the U.S. government can't stop research from happening in other countries, and this is precisely what has happened, as extensively chronicled by researcher Clint Werner in his 2011 book *Marijuana: Gateway to Health*.

"According to leading cannabis researchers Donald Abrams, M.D., and Manuel Guzman, M.D., cannabinoids seem to work against cancer through a number of different mechanisms, including killing mutated cells, slowing their growth, and preventing them from spreading or growing new blood vessels," Werner writes. "In fact, there is evidence that the cannabinoids found in marijuana have the ability to identify mutated cells, stunt their growth, cut off their blood supply, and prevent them from spreading before they can get a foothold and form tumors."

Apoptosis is a Greek term meaning "the falling away of leaves," and it describes the programmed, natural death of cells. Cancerous cells don't die as they should; instead they grow and crowd out healthy cells. Cannabinoids selectively target these cancerous cells and cause apoptosis to occur, effectively destroying malignancies while leaving healthy cells untouched. Since cannabis is a powerful anti-inflammatory, and inflammation is what causes cells to turn cancerous in the first place, it also seems as if marijuana could be used as a preventative medicine, discouraging cancer from ever manifesting.

Pro-cannabis advocates look forward to a future where research can proceed unfettered by prohibitionist politics, furthering human knowledge and the development of new medicines. If cannabis has the potential to fight cancer, then our government needs to fund wide-ranging, in-depth research toward a cure.

Indicas, Sativas, and High-End Strains

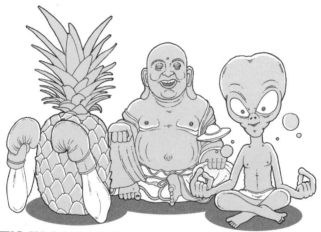

WHAT'S IN A NAME?

Due to the hard work and high-minded insights of cannabis breeders across the globe, the overall quality of marijuana worldwide has risen steadily since the first issue of *High Times* was published in 1974, with an incredible array of new varieties created along the way. So much so that an old head from that bygone era—while surely used to smoking some excellent imported *sativas* like Maui Wowie, Acapulco Gold and Thai Sticks—would nonetheless be flabbergasted if somehow transported into a modern medical marijuana dispensary, stocked with countless different varieties sporting fanciful names like Berry White, Platinum Afgoo, and Alien Thunder.

So what do these names really mean? If you track down some primo Chemdog after sampling your friend's stash, will it be the same plant with the same effects when you find it somewhere else? How much of the hype around certain strains is due to marketing versus genuine quality? And what's the best strain for me?

All good questions. Especially because the system of naming and tracking cannabis genetics is quite convoluted, with little to no oversight beyond the best efforts of magazines like *High Times*, enthusiastic online communities, and the privileged few connoisseurs able to sample enough different herb to stay on top of things.

And even then, marijuana's ongoing outlaw status makes it tough to trace a strain's true family tree with any degree of certainty. Some unscrupulous dealers will even go so far as renaming their offerings on a whim, based on whatever they think will sell the best. Even the origins of many of the most legendary strains, such as Chemdog, Cheese, Early Girl, Matanuska Thunderfuck, and Sensi Star remain shrouded in mystery. There are also lost varieties, known colloquially as "unicorns," like a mutant Orange Diesel sampled in New York City circa 2006 that tasted amazing but had unstable genetics and so failed to reproduce.

Breeding cannabis is a tricky art to master, in part because of the complicated flavors, aromas, medicinal and psychoactive effects involved, but also

IS POT STRONGER THAN IT USED TO BE?

🌿 🌿 🌿 🌿 🌿 🌿 🌿 🌿 🌿

Classic varieties like '60s era Thai Sticks, Santa Marta Gold, and Panama Red were plenty strong, otherwise no one would remember them! Pot prohibitionists like to claim that today's weed is so much stronger than the innocuous pot of the '60s, and therefore it's somehow much more harmful. In reality, the opposite is true: While average THC levels have risen over the years, users have adjusted by ingesting much less into their lungs. Which is why an old-school hippie would buy a "lid" ('60s slang for an ounce), remove the seeds, and smoke a lot of it to cop a buzz. Today we have "one-hitter quitter" herb, which reduces the amount of smoke inhaled.

because the world of marijuana remains mired in a gray or black market that holds down proper innovation. Still, we've managed to make incredible strides and produce some primo buds, with many of the top names like Haze, Kush, and Diesel becoming the stuff of pop culture legend.

BREEDING IS FUNDAMENTAL

To help understand how it all works, an analogy can be made with dog breeding, where distinct, stable genetic lines (known as purebreds) exist like poodles, cocker spaniels, and Labrador retrievers. Then there are hybrids, which come into being the first time a Labrador mates with a poodle. The resulting litter of mutts isn't immediately considered a whole new breed of dog, but in time, if you make enough mutts with this genetic cross and mate them to each other—stabilizing their genetics—you can create the Labradoodle (or a cocker spaniel-poodle cockapoo), and eventually have these dogs considered a pure breed.

A similar phenomenon takes place with cannabis, in that there are a lot of crossbreeders ("pollen-chuckers") out there making mutt hybrid plants and advertising them as a brand new kind of dog. But only a few will win the hearts of enough people to earn their place amongst the recognized pantheon of pot strains.

Continuing the analogy between man's best friend, the dog, and man's favorite plant, marijuana, we can consider the original thousands-of-years-old, wild-growing strains to be like the wild wolves that the first dogs descended from. These "landrace" varieties of cannabis adapted specifically to certain places, and typically landraces take their name from the area of their origin, like Red Congolese, Thai Stick, Afghani, Hawaiian, Panama Red, and Hindu Kush.

While not nearly as floral and flavorful as our modern hybrids, many of these landraces exhibit strong potency with an uplifting effect. They also make great breeding stock for those hoping to develop the world's next amazing new strain.

SATIVAS AND INDICAS

As we've learned, cannabis most likely originated in central Asia and spread from there all over the globe, after splitting into two distinct sub-species, with plants in equatorial areas (*sativas*) evolving to grow tall and spindly, with long, narrow leaves, and thin, wispy buds that pack a potent, uplifting,

SATIVA VS. INDICA

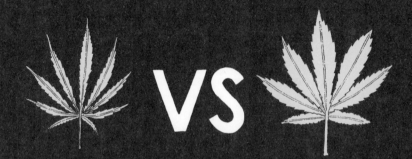

SATIVA   INDICA

SATIVA	INDICA
Energizing	Relaxing
Head high	Body stone
Promotes creativity	Promotes sleep
Helps focus	Helps pain
Fights depression	Relieves stress
Tall plants	Short shrubs
Small, loose buds	Compact, dense buds
Long flowering time	Short flowering time
Thin leaves	Fat leaves
Small yield of buds	Large yield of buds

psychedelic punch; while plants in northern or mountainous climates (*indicas*) grow shorter and stockier, with thick, wide leaves and compact, resinous buds.

Sativas take much longer to grow and yield far less than *indicas*, but remain beloved nonetheless for bestowing a soaring high that stimulates creativity and promotes activity, while *indicas* offer a body buzz that sedates and relaxes, perfect for pain relief or nighttime chilling. Some theorize that the intense sunlight absorbed by plants near the equator may account for production of more psychoactive resin in *sativa* strains.

Both sub-species produce a full range of the plant's cannabinoids, but *sativas* tend to provide more THC, which accounts for their euphoric, heart-racing properties—a highly stimulating effect fondly remembered by Vietnam vets who smoked legendary varieties like Burmese and Dalat while on their tours of duty, or anybody who ever got a hold of some Punta Roja backstage at an Allman Brothers concert. Unfortunately for cultivators, while their flowering season is long, the yield of these wispy *sativa* buds is low. And at heights of fourteen to twenty feet when fully mature, they're completely impractical for the indoor grower.

This is why it's extremely rare to find a 100 percent pure *sativa* on the market, and more common to find sativa-dominant hybrids that grow in a wider range of climates—though certain strains like Dr. Grinspoon and Neville's Haze prove that they do still exist. Also, many strains marketed as *sativas* are in fact a *sativa*-dominant hybrid, so if you're shopping at a dispensary, and you want to try a true *sativa* for yourself, don't just rely on the label. Ask someone on staff for detailed information on the plant's genetic background, such as what strains were crossed to create this particular hybrid. Or look for Red Congolese, Durban Poison or Nigerian Nightmare, a few of the most common pure *sativas* still widely available for sale.

> **"I'm more of a *sativa* guy, 'cause I work a lot. What kind of sparks what I'm working on is Blue Dream— any of them sharp-tastin', sharp-smellin' *sativas*. *Indica* makes me sleep. I don't wanna sleep and be tired; I like good energy, a good vibe."**
>
> REDMAN

Smokers seeking a pure *indica* will have a far easier time finding and growing one, since these plants flourish in most climates. Look for God Bud, Grandaddy Purps, or Blueberry for a good solid *indica* stone. *Indicas*, traditionally used to make hash, have a shorter growing season and yield more, with comparatively higher CBD levels. Fans of *indicas* revere them for their body stone, a relaxing effect that tends to "couchlock" the user, relieving pain, stress, and anxiety while easing sleep.

Growers who cross landrace *sativas* to *indicas* hope to capture the desired qualities of both in their new hybrids: a strain with an electric high that yields faster, with heavier buds and a higher yield.

DESIGNER DANK

Some of the first hybrids created from landrace *sativas* and *indicas* became classic purebred strains in their own right—legendary varieties like Northern Lights #5, Haze, or Skunk #1—as well as the building blocks of future top-shelf varieties like Jack Herer, Big Bud, and Chronic.

Legendary breeders—including Neville Schoenmaker from the Seed Bank/ Super Sativa Seed Club, Sam Skunkman and Eddie from Sacred Seeds/Cultivator's Choice, and Ben Dronkers from Sensi Seed Bank—made a name for themselves and their weed in this era, by creating the first commercially available cannabis hybrids. Skunk #1 won the first-ever *High Times* Cannabis Cup in 1988, while Sensi Seed Bank took the prize in 1994 with Jack Herer (named for the legendary activist), a combination of Skunk #1 x [Northern Lights #5 x Haze] that's still considered one of the most skillful crosses ever made due to the combination of incredible potency, amazing flavor and hefty yield.

THE ORIGINAL HAZE

The history of the classic Haze strains, with their soaring, euphoric, long-lasting highs, spicy flavors, and characteristic lanky structure, remains cloaked in legend and lore. In a work of intense stoner scholarship, *High Times* senior cultivation editor Danny Danko in his article "The Haze Craze" has managed to trace the origin of the Original Haze back to the city of Santa Cruz, circa the late 1960s: "Here, along the California coastline, the Haze Brothers cultivated an exotic variety of pot that quickly earned fame within the area's small circle of cannabis connoisseurs at that time. The

Common Strains *and* Their Characteristics

NAME	CHARACTERISTICS	EFFECT
AFGHANI #1	Fat, dark leaves and stocky growth. Dense buds are heavy with resin and exude a slight lemon odor.	Sedating, couchlock herb perfect for relaxing.
AK-47	This heavy-yielding *sativa*-dominant hybrid is popular with cultivators who grow clones.	With a very strong uplifting high, AK-47 qualifies as a one-hit wonder.
BLUEBERRY	Short, dense plants and dense buds tinged with bluish and lavender pigments.	Euphoric high with fruity flavors and complex aromas.
CHEMDOG	This incredibly aromatic diesel-fuel smelling strain requires a lot of odor control when growing.	Tangy flavor with hints of cedar and licorice.
CHOCOLOPE	*Sativa*-dominant strain takes longer to finish flowering, but it's worth the wait!	Unique chocolatey flavor from Chocolate Thai strain used as a parent.
LA CONFIDENTIAL	Compact, dark-green *indica* buds are aromatic and mold-resistant.	Interesting nutmeg flavor and an intense body high.
NEVILLE'S HAZE	Classic pure *sativa* is tall and lanky, with small buds that finishing flowering after a whopping sixteen weeks!	Inspiring, transcendent high perfect for creative and spiritual types.
PURPLE KUSH	Almost a pure *indica*, this squat plant grows purple buds.	Sweet grape flavor with a deep body stone.
ROMULAN	Short *indica* boasts purple stems and dark green leaves.	Buds have a piney aroma and peppery taste, with a pain-relieving, relaxing high.
SUPER SILVER HAZE	This multiple-Cup winning *sativa* grows tall and willowy, with thin green leaves.	Spicy dry odor complements the sweet, musky floral flavor and outstanding high.

GANJA GENETICS GLOSSARY

✹ ✹ ✹ ✹ ✹ ✹ ✹ ✹ ✹ ✹ ✹

Danny Danko's *The Official High Times Field Guide to Marijuana Strains* describes over 125 varieties, including Cannabis Cup and Top 10 Strain of the Year winners, along with commercially available strains from respected seed banks. Danko also explains the basic terminology used in discussing plant genetics.

In cases where the lineage is known, it's given with the male parent listed first (male x female: e.g., Mazar x Trainwreck). When hybrids were crossed with hybrids, they are given with the parents listed in brackets: for example, [Afghani x Kush] x [Hawaiian x Nigerian].

Cultivar	A plant variety that's been selected for desirable traits, also known in layman's terms as a "strain."
F1	The F1 or Filial 1 hybrid is the result of the first cross of two plainly different parents (i.e., a pure indica x pure sativa). These crosses typically result in hybrid vigor.
F2	A less consistent result of pollination of an F1 whose genetics will vary from good to useless.
Genotype	A particular inherited characteristic or trait, like pink hairs or purple coloration (genotype + environment = phenotype).
Hybrid	The offspring of two distinct varieties or lines.
Hybrid Vigor	Also known as Heterosis, F1 crosses with hybrid vigor improve on the genetics of their parent strains by growing stronger and quicker.
Inbred Lines (IBLs)	Genetically stable representations of a specific landrace.
Landrace	A strain that has adapted over generations to its climate and environment. Landraces show more diversity than IBLs.
Phenotype	The visible genetic expression produced by hybrids in their environment (i.e., a sativa-dominant or indica-dominant phenotype of a particular hybrid strain can be produced from the same batch of seeds).

Original Haze, rumored to contain tropical genetics from Thailand, Mexico, and Colombia, delivered an electric *sativa* jolt. The high was cerebral and uplifting, with almost no ceiling to the buzz."

Danko continues, "In the 1980s, the legendary seed producer Neville Schoenmaker bought a selection of beans from a connoisseur in New York that included the Haze Brothers' Original Haze. After he took those seeds to Amsterdam and embarked on a breeding project to stabilize them, Schoenmakers released Neville's Haze to the general cannabis-smoking public, and everything changed. As marijuana historian Mr. Haze 420 said to me, 'Neville's Haze is some of the most powerful *sativa* I've ever smoked.'

"By the end of the decade, Haze hybrids were making it easier for growers and smokers to truly appreciate the amazing qualities of the strain. Neville's Seed Bank released NL #5 x Haze in 1989, and Sensi Seeds followed shortly thereafter with their Silver Haze, winning the *High Times* Cannabis Cup that same year."

If you'd like to try a real Haze, look for Super Silver Haze from Greenhouse Seeds, Amnesia Haze from Soma's Sacred Seeds, or G-13 Haze from Barney's Farm. Haze strains come especially recommended for nausea, depression, and ADHD.

MOUNT KUSHMORE

Kush strains have become so ubiquitous that the word *kush* has actually become shorthand for "really good pot." The arrival of superior seeds from the Hindu Kush region to California in the '70s marked a time of transformation in the quality of homegrown cannabis, giving Kush "an almost mythical status as the foundation of West Coast genetics," according to Danny Danko. The psychedelic, soaring high; pungent odors of pine and lemon; wide, dark green leaves; and harvests of tight, dense little nuggets distinguish Kush varieties. Even with Kush crosses crowding the shelves of dispensaries, and getting name checked in hip-hop songs, the popularity of the O.G. Kush variety shows no signs of flagging, despite a decidedly high-minded ongoing debate over what the acronym really means (some say O.G. stands for "Ocean Grown," others say "Original Gangsta").

Cultivation editor Nico Escondido wrote about the possible origins of O.G. Kush in one of his investigative field reports: "[Its] true roots begin in the Colorado mountains, before it surfaced in a mysterious pot deal in a

GENETICS SLANG

✹ ✹ ✹ ✹ ✹ ✹ ✹ ✹ ✹ ✹

Bean	Cannabis seeds
Clone-Only	A strain that is only able to propagate through cuttings from a female plant (this is because no male plants exist for this particular phenotype)
Hermie	A hermaphrodite plant, undesirable because the genetics are unstable
Pollen-chucker	Amateur breeder
Pre-98	Marijuana genetics that existed before 1998, when over-hybridization began to muddle the gene pool

Grateful Dead parking lot. According to this legendary tale, a pound of weed was bought that contained exactly eight seeds. These were the legendary Eight Magic Beans that gave us the Chemdog, O.G. Kush, and Diesel lines, among others. Whether or not the story's completely true, tons of research by various writers has found that the herb in that deal was from an area in Colorado where a primarily *indica* Chem line had been produced steadily for years, confirming that Chemdog (and related siblings) are indeed of predominantly *indica* genetics."

Following up on the faint trail of Kush genetics, cultivation editor and strain hound Danny Danko dug even deeper in "The Story of Kush," tracing the history of this glorious cannabis back to its earliest origin.

The disputed region known as the Hindu Kush shares its boundaries with Pakistan and Afghanistan just north of Indian-controlled Jammu and Kashmir. The area has long been known for its ongoing conflicts as well as its history of cannabis and hashish production. Part of the legendary Himalayas mountain range, the fertile valleys and hillsides of the Hindu Kush have, for centuries, produced the world's finest hash. Years of natural and human selection for the most resinous, indica-dominant plants have resulted in short, stocky bushes covered with huge, shiny trichomes.

In the 1960s and early '70s, intrepid travelers on the "Hippie Trail" (including members of the Brotherhood of Eternal Love) returned to the United States, Canada, and Europe with primo seeds and began growing Afghani, Skunk, and Kush strains in earnest. Sadly, in 1973, bowing to pressure from the United States, the newly self-appointed president of Afghanistan, who took power in a bloodless coup against the long-serving and hashish-friendly Afghan king, declared the production and sale of hashish illegal. Afghan Communists overthrew the president in 1978, and the country was invaded by the Soviets in 1979, sparking another thirty years of warfare and bloodshed that continue to this day.

The Afghani hashish of the pre-war era remains legendary among older heads, and the strains that it spawned changed the cannabis growing scene completely. The indica-dominant genetics shortened typical flowering times, allowing plants to be grown all the way up to Alaska. In the process, the concept of "homegrown" changed from a term of derision to a point of pride.

Nowhere are Kush strains more prevalent than in Southern California. Many medical-marijuana dispensaries specialize in carrying as many varieties of Kush as they can get their hands on, and there are literally hundreds to choose from (OG, Larry, Tahoe, Russian Master, and Lemon come to mind). These days, there are also sativa-dominant Kushes, Purple Kushes, and "pretender" Kush strains with the name, but not the flavor or power of the true OG—but those who know can immediately discern that particular lemon-fuel odor and telltale tiny nuggets as the real deal.

Anyone looking to sample some official Kush genetics should start with Sensi Seed Bank, whose offerings include an original Hindu Kush landrace strain straight from the wilds of India. Burmese Kush from T.H. Seeds and Sour Kush from DNA Genetics also deliver the telltale tart diesel flavors and soaring high of a true Kush.

Due to their strong *indica* dominance, Kushes are recommended for chronic pain, insomnia, and stress relief.

GOING BACK TO THE LAND(RACES)

Sometime around the dawn of the new millennium, many serious pot smokers began to fear that the cannabis stock of top breeders had become degraded and over-hybridized. Many of the original traits unique to the building block varieties of Afghani, Haze, Hash Plant, and Skunk had been lost or diluted, resulting in a muddle of genetics that no one could reliably trace. This led to a huge upset at the Cannabis Cup in 2004, when a previously unknown Canadian seed breeder who went by the name of Reeferman toppled the Dutch "potocracy" by winning the highly sought after Sativa Cup with a strain called Love Potion #1. Created from landrace genetics, Love Potion was a blend of Santa Marta Colombian Gold and G-13, backcrossed to the original Colombian male to produce a smoke that blew everyone away. Reeferman had traveled and collected seeds from many remote locations, and this infusion of original genetics gave his strains incredible potency and other attributes that earned great renown.

Recently, growers have even been distinguishing their strains as "pre-98," meaning that it's an older variety with a stable genetic background. In 2011 at the Denver Medical Cannabis Cup, a pre-98 Bubba Kush from The Clinic captured the High CBD Award, with a lab-tested result of 12.7 percent CBD. Identifying strains with important medicinal qualities is part of the mission of these contests, since it's vital that cultivators preserve their high-CBD varieties for future generations. Archivists and seed savers have also been working to revive classic varieties and even resurrect vanished legends like Roadkill Skunk, once thought to be extinct.

Starting in 2010 with an expedition to Malawi, a popular documentary series, *Strain Hunters*, introduced the idea of collecting rare landrace marijuana strains to the world. Produced by Green House Seeds, Amsterdam's biggest seed company, *Strain Hunters* sends master breeders Arjan Roskam and Franco Loja to exotic locations like India, Morocco, Jamaica, and Swaziland to source wild cannabis varieties and preserve them. These landrace strains are made available to the public through the Strain Hunters Seed Bank, and the infusion of fresh genetics contributes to new breeding projects at Green House Seeds.

Breeders who make use of landrace strains are typically looking for high levels of certain medicinal cannabinoids like CBD or THCV, or they're seeking plants that grow hardier, with resistance to pests and diseases. Refreshing the cannabis gene pool insures genetic diversity and healthy thriving cannabis stocks for years to come.

SEED SALVATION

Seed saving is tremendously important to the work of heirloom growers. Just ask Mike Corral of the Wo/Men's Alliance of Medical Marijuana (WAMM), who has been refining the same four strains for over twenty years, acclimatizing his plants to the foggy weather along the Central Coast of California as part of his work with America's oldest and most compassionate cannabis collective.

Starting out in the 1970s with an African Queen *sativa* hailing from Malawi, and a Purple *indica* from Afghanistan, Corral kept the landraces going for decades, while creating both a *sativa*-dominant and *indica*-dominant hybrid cross of the two. Over the years, when deciding which plants to use for making seeds, he selects for medicinal attributes, mold resistance, and overall yield and hardiness in order to best serve the hundreds of patients who rely on WAMM medicine. The benefits of sticking with consistent genetics and refining them in this way includes being able to collect evidence of how medical marijuana helps patients, and working to determine which strains best treat specific illnesses.

As grower and *High Times* writer Anthony Luna illustrates in his article, "Landraces: A Re-Introduction," it's important to archive and catalog seeds, forming a sort of time capsule of all the varieties that were successful in the past.

"This is a very sensitive time for marijuana breeding practices," Luna writes, "as the proliferation of questionable genetics continues to dilute the species. This is of particular importance to medical marijuana patients, whose needs are focused on finding the proper medicine, not the latest hip strain. As a result, the re-emergence of landrace chemotypes is crucial to the evolution of medical cannabis."

RAISING THE BAR

Now nearing its thirtieth anniversary, The *High Times* Cannabis Cup harvest competition seeks to establish and maintain standards for the world's pot growers by awarding the field's highest honor to those who've truly mastered growing, processing, and breeding excellent cannabis. Every year, the contest ensures that new strains greet the world of cannabis connoisseurs, created by enterprising seed breeders, who hope their latest variety will bring home a trophy, or perhaps find a place in *High Times'* annual "Top 10 Strains of the Year" report.

During *High Times'* annual series of Cannabis Cup competitions at home and abroad, private panels of expert judges test marijuana flowers and hash blindly (meaning the samples are labeled only with coded numbers). Judges score the buds' appearance, aroma, taste, and potency, as well as how cleanly it burns, to assess not only the desirability of the entry's genetics, but also the skills of each grower.

When it comes to growing the finest ganja on Earth, it's not all about the seeds or clones you start with; reaching the highest ranks in this field also requires a skilled, patient, knowledgeable cultivator capable of determining what fertilizer regimen is best for an individual strain, whether to grow it in soil or a hydro system, and

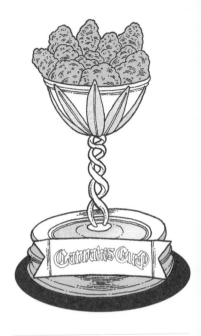

The highly-coveted Cannabis Cup.

when exactly to harvest for peak potency. (What works for *indica*-dominant Kushes won't necessarily work for *sativa*-dominant Hazes, and vice versa.)

Only a true master grower can reliably bring out the best possible representation of a particular strain. While amateurs might have great genetics and good intentions, they may fail to properly fertilize, flush, or cure their flowers, leading to a disappointing smoke.

The Cup's results are prestigious enough—as well as a trusted measure of quality—that some unscrupulous dealers claim to have the hottest new strains, such as 2013 San Francisco Cannabis Cup winners Tangelo or Girl Scout Cookies, when in reality they're peddling imposters. The key to cutting through the misinformation and marketing involves getting to know your grower, or sourcing beans from a trusted supplier and popping them yourself. Then try a blind test of different cannabis varieties to find the one that works for you without being influenced by catchy names, making an effort to include some of the classic cannabis cultivars like Skunk, Afghani, and Haze.

Invite some friends over, and it's like you're hosting your own home version of the Cannabis Cup. You'll learn a lot and have fun doing it!

How to Host Your Own CANNABIS CUP

YOU WILL NEED

grinders, filter tips, and lighters

rolling papers in different sizes for small or large joints

Pipe Wipes to clean glass and avoid germs

a variety of vaporizers and glass pieces for judges to use

microscope or magnifying glass (if you have access to one)

Anyone can throw a pot-tasting party at home with their good buddies and some good buds. While *High Times* uses a state-of-the-art digital scoring system, mathematically weighted algorithms, a panel of industry experts, and lab testing to determine the winners of our Cannabis Cup harvest competitions, simple blind tasting and basic scorekeeping can elevate any pot party into a connoisseur's contest. Have a private cannabis contest in your own backyard for 4/20, to celebrate a stoner friend's birthday, or just cause it's Friday!

You can have a contest with just a few strains, or many. Be mindful not to overload your judges with too many types of pot. You can learn a lot about tasting cannabis when only comparing three or four types, whereas trying more than ten kinds of kind bud in one night will only muddle the issue.

Appoint someone to coordinate the contest. He or she will organize and code the entries (divide the entries into separate categories for *indicas* and *sativas*) so that none of the guests/judges will know or be swayed by the true identities of the strains.

Provide each judge with a kit consisting of a few grams of each entry (identified by coded label), plus some rolling papers and smoking supplies. Each judge should grind the entry, releasing terpenes that reveal aroma and flavor. Then the herb can be rolled into joints or sampled in a pipe, bong, or vaporizer. Be sure to label the filter tips of your joints with the number of the entry so you can keep track as they go around the circle.

Have each judge evaluate the cannabis entries on appearance, aroma, taste, potency, and "burnability," and score from 1 to 5 in these categories, with 5 being the best.

- **APPEARANCE:** When examining the buds' appearance, use a microscope, jeweler's loupe, or magnifying glass to examine for mold and see if the resin glands are properly ripe, with an amber color as opposed to clear; look for any signs of hermaphrodite flowers or seeds like the small "banana" looking part of the male flower (hermaphrodites are genetically unstable and undesirable in the gene pool); plus rate the trim job. Was the bud manicured nicely, with all leaves removed? Do you see harsh leaves still attached?

- **AROMA:** This is a more subjective decision, based on how nice the ground-up bud smells. Is it fruity or flowery? Minty or piney? Make notes of the smells you notice. Fresh, well-cured buds should smell strongly of something delicious or intriguing, not like old dry grass or hay. And buds should never, ever smell moldy or mildewed.

- **TASTE:** Roll a nice, small joint from a half-gram and take a dry toke—hit the joint without it being lit. You will taste more flavors this way. Does it taste like lemons or lavender? Mangoes or pineapples? You are looking for pleasant floral, piney, spicy, or fruity tastes.

- **POTENCY:** Light your joint, hit a bong, or puff some vapor, and within two minutes you should feel the strain's effects. Only smoke a small amount so you can see if this strain is a "one-hitter quitter" or not! The "stone" or high can be very subjective, but allow at least an hour to notice how the first strain made you feel before moving on to another—otherwise it can be very difficult to discern the effects.

- **BURNABILITY:** Once you've lit the joint, observe how it burns as you smoke it. Is the ash white or gray? Does it burn evenly and smoothly? A joint with white ash that burns slowly and stays lit is a sign that the cannabis was cured correctly, whereas a harsh joint with black ash that goes out constantly can signify pot that wasn't flushed properly or cured well. Look to see if a ring of oil forms just below the joint's burning ember. The presence of that ring means pot that's high-potency and oozing with resin.

Serve water, tea, and juice-based drinks, plus put out a spread of delicious munchable appetizers. Have the judges avoid caffeine or alcohol, which can make the effects of the cannabis more difficult to judge. Keep the music upbeat and cheerful, and be sure to introduce all your judges to each other so they can compare notes. Figure on at least an hour per entry, if not two or three. Set a scheduled time when the ballots will be handed in and scores tallied. In the event of a tie, a final smoke-off between the judges is in order, and usually a frank discussion will reveal the winner. Announce the winner in a dramatic fashion, and roll up the remainder to smoke!

SCORECARD

ENTRY NUMBER	STRAIN NAME
HOW CONSUMED	JUDGE

(1 = Poor / 5 = Excellent)

APPEARANCE
1 — 2 — 3 — 4 — 5

NOTES

AROMA
1 — 2 — 3 — 4 — 5

NOTES

BURNABILITY
1 — 2 — 3 — 4 — 5

NOTES

TASTE
1 — 2 — 3 — 4 — 5

NOTES

POTENCY
1 — 2 — 3 — 4 — 5

NOTES

SCORE

/25

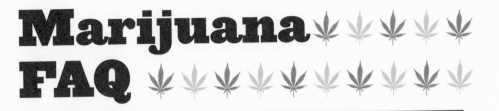

Marijuana FAQ

Dr. Mitch Earleywine has been dispensing advice to the readers of High Times *since June 2007, and is the author of* The Parent's Guide to Marijuana. *Mitch Earleywine, Ph.D. is professor of psychology at the State University of New York at Albany, and a board member of the National Organization of Reforming Marijuana Laws (NORML).*

WEED AND MEMORY My neighbor says some new study shows that using weed hurts memory even when you're not high. Is this true? —*Frank Morgan*

Hi Frank,
Australian researchers gave memory tests to almost two thousand people and found little difference between those who used the plant and those didn't (as long as folks weren't high when they were trying to learn something new). The search for a memory deficit in heavy users who aren't high at the time of the test has been so fruitless that I honestly can't imagine a need for more research in this area.

MARIJUANA AND DRIVING What's the story with fewer traffic fatalities in medical marijuana states? —*Ray Bolger*

Hi Ray,
It's true: Fatal traffic accidents drop almost 9 percent after a state passes a medical marijuana law. And after the law goes into effect, the number of alcoholic drinks consumed per person and the number of traffic accidents involving alcohol also take a meaningful drop. Looks like medical marijuana can help limit traffic deaths, and these data confirm what we've all been saying for decades: Don't drink and drive.

MARIJUANA AND MEDITATION ❧ I feel like marijuana is helping my meditation, but I wonder if it's all in my head. —*Maya*

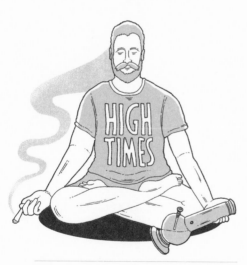

Om.

Hi Maya,

Marijuana and meditation have been linked for centuries. Many experienced users who also meditate say that marijuana can be like "training wheels" for meditation, suggesting that the plant assists in the practice. In contrast, some Transcendental Meditation fans claim that it's hard to learn to meditate if you're high, and a recent study of women who wanted to smoke less marijuana showed that they were less likely to use the plant on days when they meditated. Still, it sounds as if both can lead us to the same place.

STRAIN FOR PAIN ✔ Can you recommend a strain for pain?
—*Working Stiff*

Hi Working,
Pain is a complicated phenomenon, especially since it's manifested according to a person's biological makeup. Relaxation, regular exercise, and good sleep habits are essential for relieving pain. In terms of cannabis medicine, a moderate dose seems to have the best impact. Keep in mind, though, that high-THC strains may not work as well for pain as those with higher levels of CBD, which affects inflammation in novel ways and provides more relief. I wish we had better quality control and trademarks in the world of cannabis, but Sour Tsunami, Jamaican Lion, and Harlequin are all strains that seem to possess more CBD than average.

MANGO MOJO? ✔ Can eating mangoes make your pot more potent?
—*Popeye*

Hi Popeye,
Mangoes and cannabis both contain myrcene, a terpenoid that contributes to flavor and smell. Myrcene decreases pain and might have subjective effects similar to the "couchlock" that some folks attribute to *indicas*. Researchers haven't administered a standard dose to subjects who either have or haven't eaten mangoes, so we don't know if it really works. Fans of the practice might be unconsciously taking bigger hits or holding them longer, or they could be smoking an awesome strain called "Placebo." If myrcene really is the relevant mechanism, you'd have to eat at least four big mangoes to absorb enough of the terpene. But any healthy diet will keep you sensitive to the plant. You might as well stick with spinach.

WITCH WEED ✔ My cousin says that cannabis was part of the witches' Sabbath back in the day. Is there any truth to the idea? —*Ozzy*

Hi Ozzy,
At least one person believed that it was true: In the 1480s, Pope Innocent VIII (there's a paradoxical name for you!) condemned witchcraft and the use of hemp in what he called the "Satanic Mass." Many other plants were supposedly involved, including the hallucinogens henbane and belladonna.

Burning opium might also have been part of the rite. Certainly, it must have differed from your average church service.

DRUG TESTS AND SYNTHETIC HERB ↙ Dr. Mitch, Is there a drug test that can tell whether you've smoked synthetic herb? —KK

Hi KK,

One drug test exists that can detect metabolites for at least one of the synthetic cannabinoids (JWH-018), but it's rarely used. On the other hand, now that JWH-018 is illegal, we might see an increase in testing for it. But we know very little about these substances: They were designed for animal experiments, not for human consumption. Case studies have blamed them for causing panic and even psychosis, and the guy who first synthesized them has said that anyone who uses them recreationally is an idiot. Given the choice between a natural plant with a five-thousand-year history of safety and a chemical that was fashioned for use with rodents, which would you pick? ·

HOW DOES CANNABIDIOL WORK? ↙ I know that THC helps nausea, but does cannabidiol work, too? —Captain Diol

Hi Captain,

Cannabidiol, the non-psychoactive cannabinoid present in some strains but rather lacking in others, has many beneficial effects. New data from Canada reveal that cannabidiol alone can decrease nausea in rodents. It also appears to have a beneficial effect for those who suffer from seizures. Learn more at projectcbd.org.

DOES POT MAKE YOU SLEEPY? ↙ Does cannabis really make you sleepy, or are you just tired because it's late at night after a party? —T. Toes

Hi T.,

No, cannabis really does make you sleepy! THC sedates just about every animal that has received it in the lab, and the cannabidiol (CBD) present in many strains also increases sleep time. Even anadamide, the body's natural cannabinoid, makes mice drowsy. However, drugs that block the cannabinoid receptor CB1 have the effect of decreasing sleep time.

WEED VS. CHOLESTEROL ↙ Can marijuana fight hardening of the arteries? —R. Dahl

Hi R.,
In a research study, a small dose of THC did slow the development of cholesterol-related lesions in the arteries of mice. The effect definitely involved the CB2 receptor, which impacts the way our immune systems handle inflammation. However, I can't recommend cannabis as a cholesterol fighter. If the health benefits do generalize from mice to humans, they're probably nowhere near as significant as eating right, exercising regularly, and staying rested. But if you've got that routine down, a little help from the plant certainly wouldn't hurt.

MARIJUANA AND SENSE OF TIME ↙ I could swear you said that cannabis makes it seem time is going by faster, but I feel like it goes by slower. Which is it? —Rhythm Man

Hi RM,
That all depends on what you're doing. In laboratory studies, people reported that time does seem to pass more slowly after using the plant: For example, high folks will say that a two-second flash on a computer monitor seemed like it lasted four seconds. (Maybe that's why TV commercials and the opening credits for movies seem to go on forever.) Nevertheless, time does fly when you're having fun, so some of the results for these lab tasks—which, after all, aren't any fun—may not be applicable to other experiences.

WHY THC? ↙ Why would a plant evolve to have THC? —Chuck Darwin

Hi Chuck,
There's been a lot of crazy speculation on this subject, but one theory is that THC protects the plant and discourages predators. It definitely protects against ultraviolet rays by absorbing the sun's radiation, thereby minimizing heat damage. And THC might keep some herbivores from chomping on the leaves (much like caffeine and nicotine, which both appear to prevent certain bugs from eating various plants).

DOGGIE DOWNER? ↙ Will my dog eat my stash? —*Liza Doolittle*

Hello Liza,

Probably not—it's just too dry. But dogs love edibles as much as the rest of us. Medical marijuana states have seen an increase in the number of our best friends who have been taken to the vet with troubles related to eating brownies or cookies. So please refrigerate; you'll be glad you did. Keeping edibles away from pets is the best way to keep them healthy and save a lot of money.

WEED OF WONDER ↙ Is cannabis really the only plant in the entire world that stimulates the body's endocannabinoid system? —*Doubting T.*

Hi T.,

Cannabis is the lone plant that can alter the CB1 receptor—and in legendary ways! But caryophyllene, a cannabis compound found in black pepper, cloves, rosemary, and hops, affects the CB2 receptor. We usually think of CB2 receptors as the source of cannabis's anti-inflammatory medicinal effects. It's unclear if caryophyllene is an anti-inflammatory in people, but it seems to work in mice.

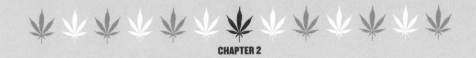

CHAPTER 2

Smoke It, Eat It, Wear It, *Be It!*

Smoke 'em if You Got 'em

HIGH ROLLER

Rolling the perfect joint is an art form practiced by stoners from around the world, and while every culture has its regional variations, there are some universal truths (it's physics, man . . .) when it comes to twisting up nice doobies. Some heads prefer glass bongs or bowls, and a few smokers will admit to an ingrained "joint-rolling disorder," (JRD) that prevents them from being confident enough in their jays to share them in a ceremonial circle. While bongs and bowls have their place, a cleanly rolled bomber allows you to taste all the flavors of your herbage much better, without being tainted by the residue that coats the inside of most pipes. If you'd like to improve your rolling and create doobies that will earn you the respect of your fellow vipers, then take heed of these vital tips:

ROLL 'EM THIN

The thinner the joint, the better the burn. Small joints, known as "pinners," have less surface area at the top where combustion is taking place. Large joints have more surface area, meaning their burn can get very hot, leading to a harsh inhale. Excessive weed in a joint can also lead to wasted smoke and more sticky resin

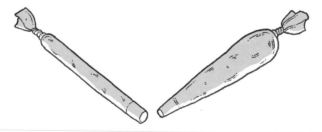

The thinner the joint, the better the burn.

accumulating at the filtered end, and getting resin in your mouth is gross. A large joint for a big circle of friends can be fun, but burning a number of smaller joints can accomplish the same goal while resulting in better flavor and appreciation of your stash. That said, the beauty of hand-rolled joints is that each one is unique, and every individual brings his or her own style and creativity to the task.

> **"Of course I know how to roll a joint."**
>
> MARTHA STEWART

THAT'S HOW WE ROLL

Rolling papers were developed in Spain for tobacco in the late 1600s, and were originally shared amongst smokers by tearing pieces from one large sheet. Papers have always been crafted from proprietary combinations of tree pulp, rice, hemp, and flax, blended to produce the desired thinness, ease of rolling, and minimal taste. The first standard size was 79 mm by 43 mm, referred to as 1¼ today. When King James enacted the world's first tobacco tax, English smokers started rolling smaller cigarettes, developing the Single Wide size. As filters became popular, papers grew larger to include them. The king was spotted smoking cigarettes rolled from papers that were 84 mm long, which became known as "King Size," but there's no official regulation of that term, so some 100 mm papers are also called King Size.

The first company to sell papers was a Spanish outfit called Pay-Pay, started in 1703. These papers were soon imitated by a French company called RizLa, and by the mid to late 1800s, brands such as Job and Zig-Zag joined their ranks. In 1894, Zig-Zag was the first to develop the "interleaving" packaging style that links one paper to the next, making dispensing papers easy. Applying the gummy "glue" to the edge of the papers was an innovation patented by RizLa in 1942, and the new inventions and improvements just keep on coming.

According to the *Denver Westword*'s pot columnist William Breathes, the brand first marketed specifically to pot tokers was the 1970s classic Randy's. This paper featured a metal wire that helped in rolling, but as the joint smoked, the wire was exposed to become a built-in roach clip. Favored by old school hippies, Randy's are still around today, although they've fallen out of fashion.

PICK A PACK OF PERFECT PAPERS

The features you're looking for in a connoisseur-quality paper are excellent burnability, ease of use in rolling, and minimal taste. Choose a non-toxic, natural adhesive such as Acacia gum. We prefer thinner hemp or rice-based papers like those produced by Raw, Bambu "Pure Hemp," or Elements, rather than thicker, bleached rolling papers containing pulp such as Zig-Zags and Clubs. Raw brand papers have become so popular that they've developed an almost cultlike following, with a wide variety of sizes made of unbleached, unrefined paper. Their patented CrissCross watermark helps keep joints burning evenly, avoiding those annoying "canoes" (a jay that burns unevenly, like a canoe shape) that happen when a joint is lit lopsided. Another newcomer to the market, boutique Jaspen papers, are also very high quality, easy to roll, and sustainably manufactured in Colorado with chlorine-free processing and all-natural Acacia gum.

TIPS ON TIPS

Filter tips have also become de rigueur for stylish smokers. While this small roll of thicker paper positioned at the end of a joint doesn't really "filter" anything, the name has stuck. Some people refer to the cardstock tips as "crutches," which have replaced the roach clips of yesteryear, and serve the same function of keeping the end of the spliff from getting too soggy. When the jay burns down to the end, simply wiggle the tip away from the herb a bit to prevent burning the cardstock while you toke the remainder. Tips make passing a

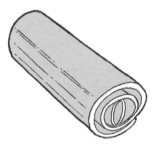

PRO TIP: Tips can keep your spliff from getting soggy.

jay easier, give you a small spot to label the strain contained within, and simply looks more aesthetically pleasing. Some types of RAW brand papers include tips, or you can fashion one from a torn business card or other cardstock.

PUT YOUR NOSE TO THE GRINDER

The grinder was a major breakthrough in stoner technology, and when the first Sweetleaf hit the market in 2000, *High Times* associate publisher Rick Cusick was there: "Inventor Joel Manson shows up in the office with a

SQUEAKY GRINDER GETS THE GREASE!

✿ ✿ ✿ ✿ ✿ ✿ ✿ ✿ ✿ ✿

When a grinder starts to get dirty, it will become caked in trichomes (those sticky crystals found coating your buds) and hard to use, either squeaking or freezing up and getting stuck when in use. If your grinder is completely frozen and stuck closed, try wiggling the edge of a butter knife in between the top and bottom piece, and continue to use the knife as a lever, moving it up and down until you work around the grinder and pop it open. Keep your grinder clean by pouring olive oil or coconut oil into each half and letting it sit overnight. Use a new toothbrush to scrub the grinder's pins, and pour all the psychoactive trichome-containing oil into a glass for later use as a drizzle of flavor to garnish a meal or a quick skin-care treatment for your dry hands or elbows.

wooden grinder and says 'This is the next roach clip!' After I tried it, I said 'I'm never going to break up a bud again without either having a grinder, or wanting a grinder.' And lo and behold, this huge brand debuted. Within months, there were hundreds of knockoffs ... "

An herb grinder consists of two pieces, a top and bottom, which form a hollow chamber lined with spikes on the inside. When the pieces are fitted together and twisted with a piece of dried plant matter in between, it breaks up the herb quickly and efficiently. Ubiquitous in India since forever, herb grinders are indispensable for rolling a perfect joint. Well-ground herb is easier to roll and results in an evenly burning joint, and avoids the time-consuming process of breaking up dense nuggets by hand, which can result in a lumpy, coarse texture and most of the resin accumulating on your fingertips. Add only a gram or so

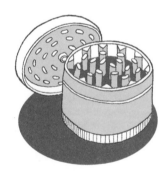

Well-ground weed results in a more even burn.

at a time, and twist the grinder. Open it up and smell the sweet aroma of freshly ground herb, before tapping the herb out onto your rolling surface. Metal grinders work better than wooden or plastic grinders, and modern grinders can be found with built-in kief screens that sift and collect trichomes and storage compartments, like those produced by Sweetleaf, Space Case, Mendo Mulchers, Bud Busters and Santa Cruz Shredders. Inventions like the MedTainer, an affordable plastic grinder and storage container, are perfect for travel.

KIEF BOXES, ROLLING TRAYS, AND POKEY-STICKS

You can roll a joint on any flat surface. We're fond of using magazines as rolling surfaces, and the subscription cards that fall out can be re-purposed into filter tips! But once you use a rolling tray, you'll never want to go back. Any simple tray will help you keep herb from falling to the floor, so look for something with sloping sides. Interesting rolling trays can be found at secondhand stores, and shallow wooden candy dishes make excellent rolling areas.

A kief box is a storage chest for your herb that contains a layer of silkscreen for sifting resin glands, collecting these trichomes on a mirror at the bottom of the box. When you break up your herb in a kief box, you are banking trichomes for future use as hash, and that's a stoner savings we can all appreciate!

One final tool will make your life much easier, and that's the humble "pokey-stick." When rolling, you frequently need a small tool to pack the herb down into the joint. An incense stick, kabob stick, or even a chopstick works wonders.

> "I used to smoke marijuana. But I'll tell you something: I would only smoke it in the late evening. Oh, occasionally the early evening, but usually the late evening—or the mid-evening. Just the early evening, mid-evening, and late evening. Occasionally, early afternoon, early mid-afternoon, or perhaps the late-mid-afternoon. Oh, sometimes the early-mid-late-early morning. . . . But never at dusk."
>
> STEVE MARTIN

STORING YOUR STASH

THC slowly converts to CBN over time, while terpenes and flavors degrade and dissipate. Old cannabis will completely dry out and appear a shade of brownish yellow. Use your cannabis within six months, and keep your pot fresher longer with these handy tips from Danny Danko:

- Avoid light and heat: store your cannabis in a cool, dark place
- Use an airtight jar, and an opaque jar for "table weed" kept out in the light
- Avoid storing pot in plastic baggies, envelopes, or aluminum foil
- Don't keep cannabis in the fridge or freezer; the humidity and cold temperatures will cause trichomes to fall off your buds

HOW TO MAKE A MUTE

Basic but effective, a mute is a paper towel tube stuffed with dryer sheets at one end. Secure one dryer sheet over the end with a rubber band, and stuff other sheets into the tube. Exhale through the one end of the tube, and your smoke emerges sweetly scented like fresh laundry. Of course, mutes won't work if you forget to use them, so stay mindful!

HOW TO ROLL: **THE CLASSIC CONE**

Commonly found in Amsterdam coffeehouses, pre-rolled cone-shaped spliffs have become popular worldwide. Avoid the pre-rolls for sale, since the pot used to stuff these is mostly dried out, stale bottom-of-the-bag shake, and roll your own from freshly ground herb to enjoy all the flavors and aromas.

1. We started with a King Size RAW paper. Add a gram of finely ground cannabis, sweeping it with your finger into a triangle shape, with more pot toward the front of the jay. Position your filter tip toward the other end.

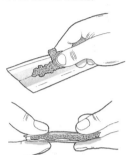

2. Tamp down the pot to get it as even as possible.

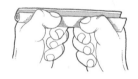

3. Tuck the paper around the filter tip at the bottom and get it tight.

4. Wrap the paper around until you see glue, then secure with a lick.

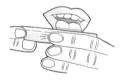

5. Fold back excess paper, over the glue. Pull paper off, starting from the bottom and moving away from you, going slowly and gently.

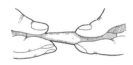

6. Tamp down by tapping filter end on the table. Use your pokey-stick to pack the open end of the jay, and scoop any fallen pot into the open end and pack it down.

7. You don't twist the top of a cone. Instead, pinch the excess paper at the top together, and shake the joint slightly. Move over finger 45 degrees and pinch and shake again. Flatten the paper so that the finished cone is flat on top. Light up and enjoy!

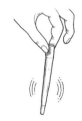

HOW TO ROLL: **THE EUROPEAN INSIDE-OUT**

Mastered by a legendary *High Times* Cannabis Cup contractor known as Thumpah Lee, this method of joint-rolling is preferred in Europe, where Thumpah learned it from a Swiss vixen. Rolling inside out allows for a tighter reefer, and you can tear off the excess paper for a cleaner taste, which is what we're all aiming for.

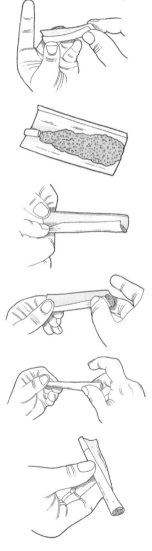

1. Take the paper (we used a King Size RAW paper) and refold the crease in the opposite direction, placing the glue side down. Position the paper with the shorter side toward you, and the glue strip to the left.

2. Roll your filter tip as tight as possible and place at the top of the paper, in the middle of the crease.

3. Grind up one gram of weed and dump onto the paper. Sort the weed into a long, thin stripe down the middle of the crease. Even out the weed with your finger and tamp it down into a tube shape.

4. Pinch the paper between your thumb and forefinger at each end and begin to roll the herb into a tube. Some weed will fall out, but that's why you have a rolling tray to catch it!

5. So you're rolling inside-out, and the glue strip is facing out. Make sure there are no creases in the glue strip; it needs to be laying flat for this to work. Begin rolling by pulling the paper tight around the filter tip and securing the glue end with your thumb.

6. With your other hand, pinch the glue to the filter as you fold the paper over the glue side and tuck the paper under. Make sure the glue stays flat and you make your way up

the joint, folding the paper tightly over and tucking as you go.

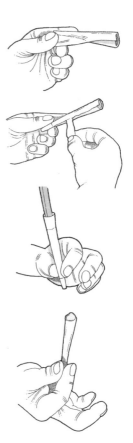

7. Roll the jay 180 degrees around until you see the glue strip under the paper. Lick along the outside paper; your saliva will soak through and adhere to the glue.

8. Run thumb and forefinger along the joint, gently pressing to make sure the glue sticks.

9. Fold back excess paper and gently tear it off from the bottom up and away from you, trying not to tear into the joint.

10. Tap filter on a solid surface to settle the herb and pack it more firmly at the open end with a pokey stick. If any herb fell into your tray, you can scrape it into a pile and scoop it back into the open end of the jay, packing it down again.

11. Twist up any loose paper at the end of the jay and shake it a bit to pack more firmly, then light it up and enjoy!

HOW TO ROLL: **THE SERPENT**

This is a favorite of *High Times'* best roller, Danny Danko, who says, "A pure pot joint with a nice thin snake of soft Moroccan hash down the middle is truly one of the finest pleasures in life." This number will knock you out with intense flavor and extreme potency. For this project you will need about .25 to .5 grams of oily hashish that's soft and pliable, preferably an import variety from Nepal, Northern India, or Afghanistan.

1. Take your hash and roll it between two non-stick surfaces, such as plastic customer reward cards or hotel key cards. (Do not use your ID or credit cards!) You can also roll the

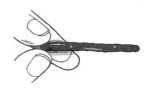

hash between your hands, since the warmth will help it soften into a thin snake just as long as your planned joint.

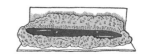

2. Prepare your joint as usual, grinding the herb and placing the filter tip. Snuggle your hash snake into the center of the herb, along the crease. You want the herb to surround the hash in the finished jay, and if the hash touches the paper, it will cause the jay to burn unevenly.

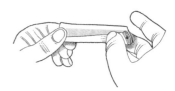

3. Take the paper between your thumb and forefinger on each side. Roll the herb into a tube shape, checking to make sure the hash has remained in the center.

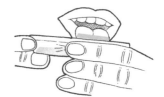

4. Tuck the non-glue edge under and wrap the glue strip over the paper, pulling it tighter and securing with a quick lick.

5. Tamp the filter end against a hard surface, and pack down the open end gently, adding any herb that fell out. Twist up the excess paper at the top and prepare to get blazed!

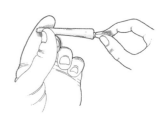

HOW TO ROLL: DOUBLE BARREL

This is a joint for when you want to double your fun! Trick joints like this use creative techniques to create more elaborate shapes. For instance, cutting the glue strip off another paper is an excellent way to secure multiple papers together, or seal joints when they tear.

1. Start with two regular joints, rolled about 10 mm in circumference. Place the two jays together, side-by-side, and wrap the filters in an extra wide filter, which you can secure by using a torn off gum strip from another paper.

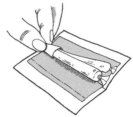

2. Wrap the joint in an extra-large King Size paper, squeezing the two joints tightly together. Use a scissor to trim off the excess paper and tips of the two original jays, and prepare to blast off with one super-smoke!

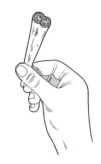

HOW TO ROLL: TRAILER PARK BOYS' SIX-PAPER JOINT

The hit Canadian TV show *Trailer Park Boys* features a series of misadventures perpetrated by a crew of low-class petty criminals in a trailer park who are always in and out of jail. Ricky, Bubbles, and Julian are usually growing weed, shooting guns, getting "drunk as fuck" and evading the park supervisor Jim Lahey.

High Times was lucky enough to sit down and puff with these hilarious actors, and the experience was captured in a YouTube video, "Trailer Park Boys in Six Paper Joint." Julian starts by saying, "I've rolled up quite a few joints in my day, especially in jail. Great dope in jail—it's expensive though." As he proceeds to roll the masterpiece, Bubbles keeps chiding him, "What's taking so long? It would be nice to get baked sometime today!" and finally Ricky has to step in and assess the finished jay, saying, "You should have let me roll this, man, you fucked up. But I'll smoke it anyway." And that's really the point here. Even if your joints aren't pretty, as long as they function, you're good to go!

1. Start with six papers: 1¼ size is just fine (King Size may become unwieldy). Begin by creating a giant paper by using the gum to attach the papers to each other, two papers wide and three papers long. Secure the sides without glue strips by cutting glue strips from another few papers and using those to attach the short sides together. Wet your finger and run your finger over the glue strips; this will get them to adhere.

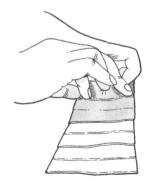

2. Grind 7 to 10 grams of weed and dump into center of the giant paper. Use your finger to nudge herb into a long, thin pile. Position a 32 mm filter (cut from an old business card) at the bottom end of the huge jay.

3. Pick up the jay at either end and begin to gently roll and massage it into shape.

4. When the herb is sufficiently rolled, tuck the non-glue edge over the herb and pick the gum on the top paper. Seal the top paper over the bottom, tightening as you go.

5. Use a pencil or pen to gently pack the herb down from the open end. Twist up the remaining paper and light it up!

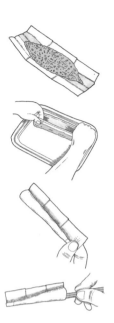

HOW TO ROLL: **THE CALI-CANNON**

Our amazing photographer Lochfoot shared an insane joint-rolling method in our February 2013 issue. Since we've never seen an equal to this Sonoma cigar, we'd like to enshrine this mega-doobie in the *High Times* Joint-Rolling Hall of Fame. Try it if you dare!

Lochfoot writes:

You'll need the better part of an eighth to build this mother, and trying to smoke it down with less than three heads is suicidal. Some jumbo-size papers will also be required. And if you don't have Andre the Giant–sized hands, you will need either a dollar bill or, in our case, a well-used playing card from an old deck to keep things even. Finally, while the Cali-Cannon is good to the last puff, it's also a good idea to use a crutch, which you can make from another card (believe me, the deck you've sacrificed will forgive you).

The master recipe also calls for at least 2 grams of the finest hash you can get your sticky little hands on—and remember not to insult the strain with a substandard chunk of hardened goo from some novice basement producer. Accompanying the fine hash will be its viscous counterpart, known to many as honey oil—just enough to coat the last inch of the cannon. Last but not least, you'll need a pinch of pure kief to roll onto the honey-oil end and help blast you off into space.

1. Now that you've got the ingredients together, start off by breaking down your herb into joint-rolling consistency, remembering to remove any stems that might tear a hole in the mothership.

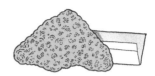

2. Warm up the hash a little by gently squishing it between your palms until it has the consistency of Play-Doh. The idea here is to roll it into a thin shaft that will run the length of your Cali-Cannon.

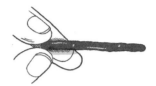

3. Now it's time to roll. Place your ground greenery inside the paper on top of the rolling card. Next, lay the hash shaft down the center of your pile with the crutch on one end and then roll away. Take your time and remember: It requires some practice to master this particular technique. Keep some extra papers on hand to repair any minor holes or splits along the way.

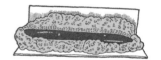

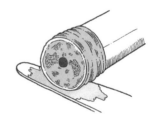

4. Once your joint is rolled, it's time to apply the honey oil to the end of the barrel. Here, we gooped the oil onto a butter knife and gently rolled the bomber 360 degrees for an even coat.

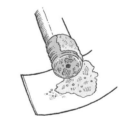

5. Finally, we placed our kief onto the playing card that we fashioned into a crutch and dredged the end of our Cali-Cannon through the mind-numbing powder as the finishing touch.

6. Now it's go time . . . put on your tunes of choice, fire this sucka up, and initiate liftoff!

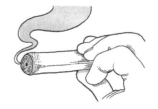

BUD TRIMMING TIPS

Prepare your trimming room with a clean table, plenty of small scissors, and some comfortable chairs. Anyone you have helping out must be a trusted friend. Make sure they understand the importance of keeping quiet about your operation. Your security, as well as theirs, depends on resisting any urge to brag about the work being done. It'll take one experienced trimmer about two to four hours per pound, so choose helpers wisely (if you need them at all).

Use sharp pruning clippers to cut the plant at its base. Trim plants whole or cut them into easier-to-manage branches. The goal is to remove the fan leaves and trim any secondary leaves that stick out from the buds and don't have many resin glands on them. The closer to the flowers you trim, the less leaf you'll be smoking later, so take your time. Use these leaf trimmings to make dry or water-extracted hash and cannabutter.

Periodically, clean your trimming equipment; that's the time to take a break and try some "scissor hash." Before you scrub the scissors with rubbing alcohol and a rag or paper towel, scrape the sticky residue off and pack a bowl. This is some of the strongest and spiciest smoke you'll ever try; it makes all the meticulous and sometimes boring busywork more fun. Stay vigilant and keep these breaks short; they have a tendency to extend further than planned.

Always hang your plants to dry in a dark room or closet. Humidity levels in the drying area should be approximately 50 percent to 60 percent and the temperature should be between 60°F and 70°F. Have a fan circulating air in the room but not directly blowing on the plants. Within four to seven days, the buds will be crispy on the outside and ready to begin the curing process.

If you choose to cut individual branches, you can use them as hangers as well, eliminating the need for ties or clothespins. Each branch becomes its own hook to hang on the drying line. Make sure not to crowd the branches too close together; air movement around the buds reduces the risk of mold.

Some people reverse the trimming and drying process and hang their plants without manicuring them at all. They trim the leaves off the buds after drying the plants whole. This may be a bit more time-consuming but the finished product inevitably dries slower, and slow drying makes for tastier pot.

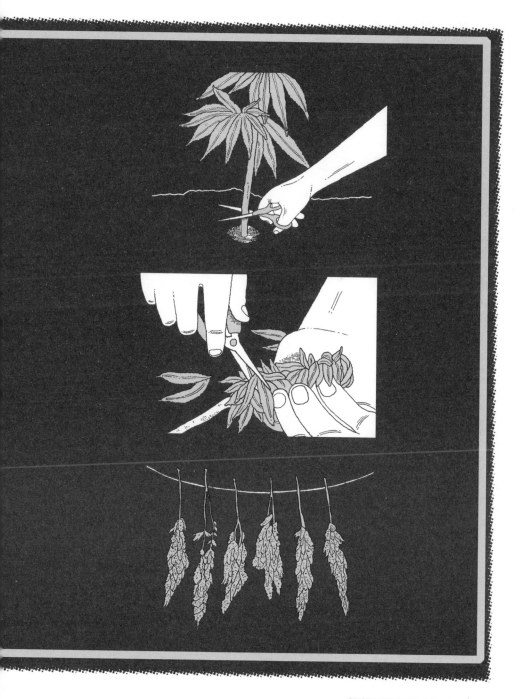

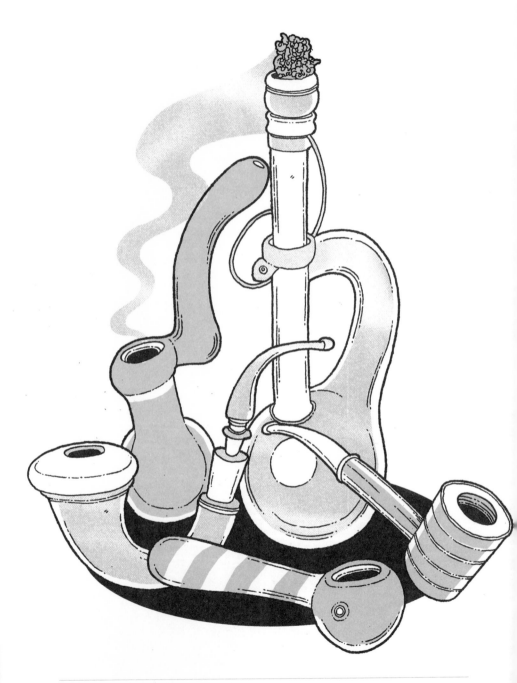

Glass act.

Head *of* the Glass

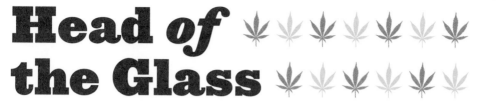

WHERE DO BONGS COME FROM?

Many marijuana enthusiasts form a special connection with their glass pipe, which makes sense, since such a treasured tool—used in so many special herb-smoking rituals—becomes associated with relaxation, positive energy, and good vibes in the extreme for all who cross its path. But where do these implements come from?

Early bongs were made of hollow gourds or ceramics, much like the artifacts discovered in Ethiopian caves that date back to 1320. In museums worldwide, you can see antique pipes (intended for tobacco use only, or so they say!) carved from bone or horn, wood or stone. The extensive paraphernalia collection of Michael and Michelle Aldrich, cannabis activists in San Francisco, includes early '60s bongs made from hollow bamboo tubes, African pipes of wood and metal, and creative oddities like early honey bear bongs. Semi-disposable corncob pipes can still be found in liquor stores, and before the glass pipe movement took hold, most heads in the '60s were puffing from pipes made of metal or wood.

The evolution of glass pipe art in North America is actually a fascinating story, starting with hippies like Bob Snodgrass, a pioneer in borosilicate glass work who traveled on Dead tour selling smoking paraphernalia to fellow weed-loving wanderers. Responsible for innovations like creating color-changing glass that shifts tones as the pipe gathers resin, Snodgrass is credited as the father of the glass pipe art movement. Speaking to *High Times* in a 2006 interview, he recalled, "In 1972, I was experimenting with putting different powdered metals into the glass . . . we discovered copper reds and copper greens. I also found that silver and gold could be blended and sprayed onto the glass. A new technique of spraying metals into glass changed the parameters of color possibilities."

Snodgrass, headquartered in Eugene, Oregon, began educating many young glassblowers throughout the '80s and by the 1990s, legions of Snodgrass acolytes hawked their wares on Phish tour, selling pipes in parking lots. Headshops caught on and began carrying artistic glass pipes, and as the internet matured, online retailers made original glass art available nationwide. Business boomed, and thousands of people embarked on careers blowing glass.

With the rise of dab culture (see page 115) requiring new paraphernalia to handle sticky, gooey cannabis concentrates, innovations have fueled a renaissance in high-quality art glass, as up-and-coming artists capture the imaginations of a new generation of heads with innovative oil rigs, bongs, and pipes. New outfits like Hitman Glass have captured the creativity of underground glassblowers with ambitious projects like *Chess Pieces*, wherein artists were invited to create a high-art chess set that's also a functional smoking piece, with the results featured in a gallery show and a lavish art book.

Largely sparked by dab culture, this new wave of innovation in glassware, with artists such as Zach Puchowitz, Banjo, Eusheen, Ryan "Buck" Harris, and Darby Holm continuing to push the boundaries. Amongst young dabbers, master glass blowers command the same kind of respect and recognition as rock stars and pro skateboarders, with outfits like the Mothership establishing a cult of devoted followers. Stylish new glass galleries such as Gathering Glass, Mary Jane's House of Glass, and Easy Street Gallery feature all-American, handmade pieces that cater to and support this new market for high-end, locally blown glass.

SELECTING THE PERFECT PIPE

Glass can be a big investment, so take getting a new pipe seriously. We suggest buying in person, which will allow you to touch and test pipes (inhaling air) before you buy, which is impossible online. Patronize local headshops, and comparison shop to see who has the best pieces and the best vibe.

Usually, when you're browsing in the store, a certain piece will call out to you. Ask to hold it and see how it fits in your hand, and you'll know instinctively if it feels right. Take a practice inhale so you can test how the air flows through the pipe. Look for any chips or cracks that could cause the piece to break. Examine the bowl and carb for rough edges, which are evidence of drilling. An imported pipe must have the bowl hole and carb drilled into

THE WAR ON PIPES

In February 2003, fifty-five glass-blowers and several major companies were targeted for their deviant art by the DEA's Operation Pipe Dreams, which took down Chong Glass, Jerome Baker, 101 North, Sunshine Distribution and others for violations of federal law related to selling paraphernalia over the Internet. Tommy Chong ended up serving nine months in jail, while others lost their businesses and life savings. Ken, owner of Chameleon Glass, told *High Times* in 2008, "After Pipe Dreams, good-paying blue-collar glassblowing jobs nearly disappeared, along with domestic manufacturers. And with them went a wealth of innovation capability in function and design." Slowly, business rebounded, and today you can find online headshops doing business in a legal gray area.

it after arriving in the United States, resulting in powdered glass shards remaining to be inhaled and possibly cause lung damage. Support local glass artists, and ask the store if they carry imported pieces so you'll know what to avoid.

One important consideration is whether to chose a wet piece or a dry piece. Wet pieces like bubblers or bongs use water for filtration and to cool the smoke, but they can also spill stinky water all over. Be sure all wet pieces have study bases so they won't tip. Dry pieces are much easier to transport.

Pipes called Sherlocks have a curving stem, styled much like the pipe that Sherlock Holmes would've used. Pipes with long, thin stems have also become known as Gandalfs, after the pipe used for puffing Halflings' Leaf in *The Lord of the Rings* movies. Sidecars are pipes with the bowl jutting out to the side. If you're considering a fanciful pipe with a complicated, curvy design with many long bends or multiple chambers, think about how easy it will be to clean. Are openings wide enough to pass a pipe cleaner through?

INVESTING IN AN OIL RIG

If you're purchasing a bong or oil rig, consider how and where you will be using it. Infrequent use versus constant use, portability versus style, and a tight budget versus an unlimited bankroll will determine the type of piece that you pick.

Examine the fittings where the bowl and tube come together. If the fittings are glass-on-glass, check to make sure they fit correctly and form a proper seal. If you're looking at oil rigs, make sure the mouthpiece is angled far enough away from the nail to protect your face in case of a flare-up from a bad dab. The telltale sign of quality glassware is weight. A professional piece should be heavy, while cheap knockoffs are lightweight to the point of eggshell fragility.

While many cannabis consumers find the various features of scientific glass waterpipes and oil rigs to be fascinating, those who haven't been following the glass subculture can feel intimidated by all the jargon. Many newer water pipes and oil rigs are designed with filtration devices inside known as percolators, which come in many different styles such as "honeycomb" and "showerhead." Percolators run the smoke through the water to break it up and cool it down. For smoking flowers, invest in a fancy percolation system because flowers create more tar and smoke than concentrates.

For those purchasing an oil rig, percolators are more for flash and less for function. You don't want to percolate your dab hit too much, or you lose flavor. A small "perc" is enough to cool the average dab hit.

NAILED IT!

Sean Black, marijuana activist and concentrate expert, advises would-be dabbers to remember that the nail used for smoking extracts is actually more important than the glass rig it's attached to. "Make sure to get T2 medical grade titanium," Sean explains, "and make sure you find a reputable, trusted supplier."

Unscrupulous dealers will sell metal nails made of mixed alloys, which are not made to withstand the high heat from a blowtorch and will deteriorate and flake over time. It's virtually impossible to tell if a nail is made of T2 titanium just by looking at it, but cheap nails made with alloys will be magnetic, whereas titanium is not. Those who want the purest taste from their BHO also favor quartz nails, since these crystal nails don't deteriorate like metal, but they can be fragile and costly.

KEEP YOUR PIECE CLEAN

No one wants to smoke bowls from a nasty, resin-clogged pipe. Keep your glassware looking its best by cleaning it regularly. Here's how:

WHAT YOU NEED

hot water

clean earplugs or a sponge

isopropyl alcohol

rock salt

lemon juice

1. Let hot water run through your piece until it's almost scalding.

2. Plug the holes in the piece with new foam earplugs or cut pieces of sponge.

3. Fill the glass piece one-quarter full of hot water and add enough isopropyl alcohol to bring the level of liquid inside to about half of the glass's volume. Add several pinches of rock salt.

4. Agitate the glass to swirl the solution around inside, and then let it sit for several hours. (Avoid an overnight soak in isopropyl, as it can remove color from glass if left in too long.)

5. Dump the solution. Add another round of hot water, alcohol, and salt if desired. If resin still coats the inside, try adding a higher proportion of isopropyl and soaking longer. You can also try gently scrubbing with a new toothbrush or pipe cleaner if necessary, but be careful.

6. After most resin is removed, rinse the glass with more hot water and lemon juice to remove any chemical residue and odor.

For expensive glass paraphernalia, don't even risk shaking—spring for a store-bought solution such as Formula 420 or Kush Clean that will allow you to clean the piece by soaking and rinsing only.

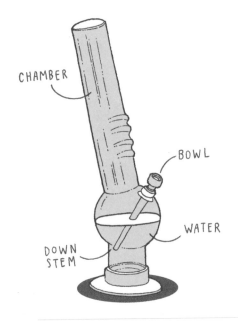

CHAMBER

BOWL

WATER

DOWN STEM

The bong.

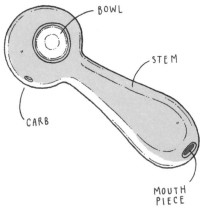

BOWL

STEM

CARB

MOUTH PIECE

The pipe.

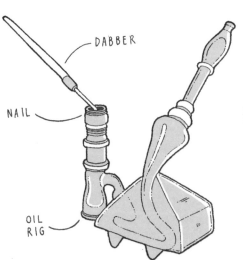

DABBER

NAIL

OIL RIG

The oil rig (a bong for concentrates).

GLASS GLOSSARY

✲✲✲✲✲✲✲✲✲✲✲

Borosilicate	Very sturdy glass that is heated to a much higher temperature than other types of glass, resulting in pipes that are more durable.
Bubbler	A wet piece shaped more like a traditional pipe than a bong, bubblers have a bowl, down stem, water chamber, and mouthpiece all in one design. They include chubblers, sidecars, Sherlocks, and hammers.
Carb	This hole in the glass regulates airflow. Cover it with your finger while inhaling, let the pipe fill with smoke, then open the carb to send fresh air rushing in, which will clear the smoke into your lungs in seconds.
Chillum	Originally from India, this is a straight cylinder tube with bowl on one end. Simply pack it and clasp between your hands to inhale.
Dichro	Short for Dichroic, this metallic coating added to glass reflects and refracts light, resulting in a shimmering, glittery color.
Diffuser	Multiple holes in the bottom of the down stem of a bong or oil rig.
Dry Piece	A smoking device that doesn't use any water filtration, including chillums, steamrollers, spoons, hammers, Sherlocks, and sidecars.
Glass on Glass	When ground glass joints are used to join the various pieces of a bong or oil rig; a setup that's superior to rubber grommets.
Inside Out	Color is applied to the inside of the pipe, where it shines vibrantly through the clear outside layer of glass.
Marble	A globe of blown glass with a variety of decorative patterns and designs inside that's either fused to a pipe or left freestanding.
Percolator	An extra chamber that allows smoke to be further filtered by water.
Slide/Bowl	A bowl that can be filled with herb, smoked, then slid out of a waterpipe to send air through the opening left behind, clearing the smoke.
Steamroller	A large, cylindrical dry piece with a bowl in the middle and openings at each end.
Spoon	A simple style of dry pipe shaped similarly to a spoon.
Wet Piece	Any smoking device with built-in water filtration, including bongs, oil rigs and bubblers.

Paraphernalia Pros and Cons

Trying to decide what you should pack for a trip out? This handy chart will help you compare the advantages and disadvantages of various devices designed for smoking or vaporizing.

	DISCREET	EFFECTIVE	PORTABLE	PERFECT FOR:
LARGE GLASS BONG	Is that a foot-long bong in your pocket? Or is it a sandwich?	Nothing packs a wallop quite like a big bonghit!	It's not easy to transport or conceal a bong, plus it could get broken.	Reigning over the living room table, safe at home.
SMALL PIPE	Easier to hide than a bong, but still not stealthy.	Sometimes a nice bowl just hits the spot!	Make sure to keep it in a padded bag to conceal the smell!	Hiking or camping trips, somewhere without a lot of people.
JOINT	It's hard to tell if you're smoking a jay or a cigarette from a distance.	Depending on how large you roll them, joints deliver a soaring high for a solo stoner or a crowd.	Rolling up a bunch of joints and storing in a tin or empty cigarette box is the way to go!	Anywhere, except places where the excessive smoke and smell might draw attention.
VAPOR PEN	Looks just like an e-cigarette, so it's easier to conceal.	You won't get as blazed as with a joint, but you can maintain a level high by sipping on it occasionally.	This is how James Bond would get baked. Nothing's more portable than a slim vapor pen.	Airports, churches, hospitals, PTA meetings, company picnics, weddings of your relatives.
VOLCANO VAPORIZER	Are you kidding me? It's pretty hard to explain away a bag of vapor.	Volcano vapor is smooth, flavorful and long-lasting for a superb high.	Since it plugs in, it's not too easy to bring the Volcano to a festival, but it has been done!	The bedside table. You can even use the vapor bag as a pillow! Sweet dreams!

HOW TO BUILD: BOTTLE BONG

For all the budding "stoner MacGyvers" out there worried about what happens if you get stuck somewhere with no pipes, bongs, bowls, blunts, or rolling papers and want to get high, we proudly present ingenious options for crafting quality smokeware out of recycled and repurposed materials—even groceries will do in a pinch! Just remember, homemade bongs or pipes should be considered a temporary solution, since using aluminum foil or plastics for smoking devices isn't healthy in the long-term.

Find more homemade smoking devices, seek out a copy of Randy Stratton's classic shopclass/kitchen table stoner how-to *Build This Bong*.

YOU WILL NEED

empty bottle from a 16-oz or 1 liter drink

pen

aluminum foil

(These items are easy to find at hotels or restaurants, making this project suitable for travelers)

X-Acto knife, Swiss Army knife, or small, sharp scissors

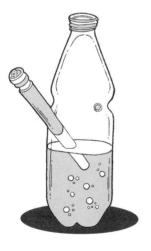

1. Take pen apart, unscrewing the nib and removing the ballpoint and ink cartridge, keeping the empty tube, which you will use as a down stem.

2. Cut a piece of foil two inches square. Take the bottle cap or your finger and hold it against the end of the pen. Wrap the foil around both the cap and the pen, molding the shape of the foil against the area where the two pieces meet. Remove the bottle cap (or finger) and you can see the foil forms the rough shape of a bowl.

3. Cut a square of foil a few layers thick, and use it to form a bowl, pushing it down into the center of the depression and folding the edges down over the lip. Poke a few holes in the bottom of the bowl. Slide the entire foil stem up the pen a few inches to avoid melting the plastic pen.

4. Cut one hole a few inches from the bottom of the bottle, slightly smaller than the pen stem. Cut a second hole on the other side of the bottle a few inches from the top—this will be your carb. Fit the pen stem into the hole and angle it toward the bottom of the bottle. Fill the bottle with water until the end of the stem is submerged.

5. Ta-da! You are ready to smoke in a survival situation. Just get yourself to a headshop as soon as possible to purchase a more suitable smoking system!

HOW TO BUILD: APPLE PIPE

It's comforting to know that if you ever break your three-foot, double-chamber, dragon-shaped glass pipe, you can always use a Bic pen and an apple to craft a fully functional replacement. Smoke from the forbidden fruit when you're on the road, at the beach, visiting Grandma, or anywhere else you don't have access to your usual arsenal of pot paraphernalia. In fact, why stop with just one edible implement, when you can smoke an apple pipe for knowledge, a carrot to treat cataracts, and a potato for St. Patrick's Day? And when you're done, simply take a bite out of crime, and swallow the evidence.

YOU WILL NEED

apple

disposable pen, such as a Bic

knife

1. Remove the ink from a disposable pen so you have a small plastic tube with nothing inside.

2. Jam the pen halfway into the apple at a shallow angle. Start near the core where it's easiest to push it in. This will eventually be your bowl.

3. On the opposite side of the apple, poke another hole that meets up with the first. This is where your lips will go.

4. Poke another connecting hole closer to the bowl, which will serve as a carb. Keep your finger over the carb when you light the bowl and then release your finger to clear the smoke in the pipe.

5. Use a knife to carve out the bowl deep enough to hold at least one solid hit's worth of weed, and start smoking!

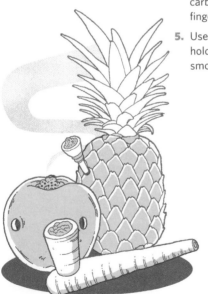

Vaporize It

(And Don't Criticize It)

DEEP BREATH

The healthiest and most discreet method of inhaling the plant's essential oils and intoxicating compounds, vaporization works by heating marijuana until its psychoactive elements boil off into a vapor that the user inhales. Some tabletop models use a large bag to capture this vapor, which is then removed from the device and inhaled through a mouthpiece, while other designs deliver vapor through a tube or straw. Enthusiastic users report a clearer, longer-lasting high and an unbeatable taste, since there's no smoke to cover over the aroma and flavor of the buds' terpenes and flavonoids.

Vaporizers also tend to use less marijuana to achieve the desired result, so those on a budget get more bang for their buck. You can even use the almost exhausted plant matter, called dottle, that's left over after vaporizing to make edibles.

Using a vaporizer is the most efficient way to ingest healing cannabinoids, and using a vaporizer is important for those concerned about the health effects of smoking. While a 2012 study published by the *Journal of the American Medical Association* found that people who smoke only cannabis have less risk of developing lung cancer than non-smokers who don't use tobacco or cannabis, reducing the amount of burning particulate matter that goes into your lungs is undoubtedly a benefit. Researchers theorize that the protective cannabinoids shield the body from the harms of inhaling toxic compounds like polycyclic aromatic hydrocarbons, benzopyrene, nitromosines, and carbon monoxide created by combusting vegetable matter. Sponsored by the Multidisciplinary Association for Psychedelic Studies (MAPS) and California NORML, a 2000 study found that vaporization produced a higher cannabinoid-to-tar ratio than joints, which produce ten times more tar than cannabinoids.

WHO INVENTED VAPORIZING?

🍁 🍁 🍁 🍁 🍁 🍁 🍁 🍁 🍁 🍁

High Times has been following the development of this useful technology from the very beginning, when a mysterious individual called Dr. Lunglife delivered a manuscript to the office describing how to build a DIY vaporizer out of parts found at RadioShack. Entitled "Vaporizing THC Oil: An Alternative to Smoking Marijuana," the first article detailing Dr. Lunglife's theories was printed in our May 1989 issue. In 2004, longtime editor Steven Hager published "The Revolution Will Be Vaporized," including a detailed description of how Dr. Lunglife turned people on not only to the idea of vaporizing, but also to making hash oil—a highly concentrated form of cannabis:

"With vaporization, Dr. Lunglife explained, the essential THC oil is heated just enough to melt the active ingredients and transform them into smokeless vapor. If there's no fire, smoke, or combustion, he concluded, there are no cancer-causing gases or tar.

"Dr. Lunglife advocated a two-step process: First, he made concentrated black oil from raw cannabis flowers, thus eliminating the plant material in stage one. He then brushed the oil onto the filament of a small lightbulb, which would be momentarily heated to complete the vaporization process. Seven months later, in the December 1989 issue, Dr. Lunglife published instructions ("Dr. Lunglife Invents a Better Vaporizer") on how to build an improved version that included a dome cover and had the capability to vaporize raw plant material."

Hager also relates the tale of Eagle Bill, a much-loved character who worked for Sensi Seeds in Amsterdam. Beginning at the seventh annual Cannabis Cup in 1994, Eagle Bill would stand at a booth all day and let visitors sample the vapor coming from his homemade contraption.

"Eagle Bill utilized a heat gun with temperature control and a large glass receptacle to contain the vapors." Hager writes, "Using mostly bottom buds and trim leaves, he demonstrated how shake could yield a pure, clean high as powerful as any produced by a joint of kind bud. Over the years, thanks to Eagle Bill, thousands of smokers experienced their first vaporization at the Cannabis Cup."

When researching the many different types of vaporizers on the market today, it's important to consider your budget and your needs. Many people who use marijuana for medical purposes favor the Volcano vaporizer, which is highly regarded for its quality engineering and reliability, but carries a hefty price tag. Other people favor the discreet vapor pens that dominate the scene today, since these devices are more affordable, portable, and easier to conceal than a large tabletop unit like the Volcano. Be sure your chosen vaporizer has a precision temperature-control method, since THC boils off at 314°F and CBD at 356°F. Whatever device you favor, be sure to look for reviews online and see if the manufacturer covers your purchase with a warranty. Make sure the company selling the vaporizer has an established reputation and has been in business for several years. So many new vaporizers have entered the market that *High Times* publishes an annual review of the best products.

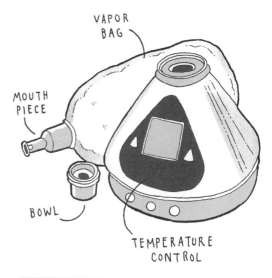

VAPOR BAG

MOUTH PIECE

BOWL

TEMPERATURE CONTROL

The vaporizer.

THE VAPOR PEN IS MIGHTIER THAN THE JOINT

With the advent of discreet, hand-held vapor pens that mimic e-cigarettes, vaporizing marijuana has almost gone mainstream. You probably even know somebody who does it regularly, or have seen folks around town pulling on a futuristic-looking gadget that enables them to sip on the vapor of cannabis flowers or hash oil without attracting any unwanted attention.

For ailing patients and dedicated stoners alike, vapor pens make taking a sneaky puff far easier than ever before, including in places like restaurants and offices where you'd never, ever blaze up a spliff. These devices can be expensive and tricky to operate, however, so *High Times* tests the best models on the market annually, publishing our recommendations online for all to see.

New models are released all the time, but the basics of how these devices operate is usually the same. Most vapor pens work by filling a small chamber with hash or ground bud, screwing the cap back on, and pressing a small button for a few seconds to heat the material. Then you draw on the end of the device, sipping in vapor and inhaling it.

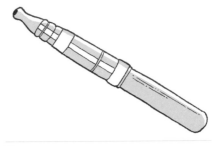

The vapor pen.

Convection and conduction are the two heating methods generally used for vaporizing. During convection heating, the vegetable matter or oil never makes direct contact with the heating element, rather, it's mixed in a "polyfill" medium. Hot air passes through this medium, which is held in a cartridge, until the vapor is released.

Conduction heating works when a substance is heated by direct contact with a metal element. Generally consisting of a wick (usually silica) and a metal filament or coil (made of nickel, aluminum, or steel), these types of vaporizers are often encased in a small bowl (typically ceramic) and centered inside a chamber or tank.

If you see a vapor pen package marked "glycerin only," this means it's designed only for cannabis concentrates dissolved in a base solution like propylene glycol or vegetable glycerin that acts as a water-attracting component, to facilitate vaporizing the solution once it's hot enough.

If you dry-burn a conduction-type vapor pen, they may produce smoke, so it's helpful to first saturate the wick with concentrate, either by applying a dab and letting it drip down, or filling the tank with solution. You may also need to pry off a small plastic lid, which is used to contain the glycerin solution, to access the tank. Leave the plastic lid off if you're using more solid concentrates such as wax or budder.

Many vapor pens look extremely similar, have interchangeable parts and chargers, and even operate from the same base unit powered by a lithium ion battery. These "standard units" are largely manufactured in China, and have been approved by the FDA for use with nicotine in e-cigarettes. Be sure to fully read the instructions before operating any vapor pen to guarantee safe and effective usage, and always fully charge the battery unit before you use it for the first time to establish long life.

Hash, Concentrates, and Extracts

HASH TRADITIONS

Hash is simply the collected psychoactive crystals from the surface of the marijuana plant, pressed together to form a ball, slab, or disc. For nearly a thousand years, hash has been made with sieves that separate marijuana's oil-filled trichomes, or resin glands, from surrounding plant matter. In countries like Morocco, where these traditional methods remain the norm, freshly harvested crops are typically left to dry in a cool, dark, well-ventilated place, curing for up to a month. Then, when it's time to collect the resin, hashmakers stretch silk scarves or other porous fabric over washbasins and place the dried buds on top. A layer of sheeting is draped over the cannabis and the basin. The sheeting is then beaten with a stick, knocking the trichomes through the sieve and into the basin (the sheeting prevents the resin from floating into the air). The collected powder, known as kief, can be consumed in this form, as raw, loose granules, or be pressed into hash. Other traditional methods of

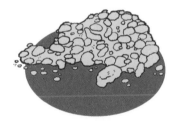

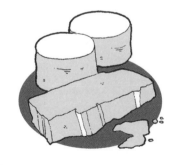

Hash, unpressed and pressed.

hash-making include hand-rubbing, where resin is collected by hand directly from live plants and rolled into fragrant balls, and carpet collection, where plants are beaten against specially woven carpets.

As extensively documented in Robert Connell Clarke's classic tome *Hashish!*, hash has a long history throughout the Middle East and Southeast Asia, in places like India, Nepal, Pakistan, Afghanistan, Turkey, Greece, Egypt, Lebanon, and Syria. In the late 1960s and early 1970s, during the glory days of the so-called "Hippie Trail," travelers could pass overland from Europe, through Istanbul, then onward to famous hash-producing towns like Chitral, Kashmir, and Manali, before ending up on "Freak Street" in Kathmandu, where spheres of psychoactive resin called Nepalese temple balls were sold openly at hashish shops.

Some heads brought their stashes down to the beaches of Goa, where hippies escaped the harsh mountain winters. Old freaks still reminisce about the golden age of Afghan hash, which had a characteristic taste and smell that distinguished it above all others.

Naturally, some of those hippies couldn't resist bringing a souvenir home. Besides being inexpensive, compact blocks of hash were far more potent and easier to conceal than marijuana. The Brotherhood of Eternal Love, a group of psychedelic visionaries composed of California surfers, bikers, and freaks, famously started smuggling kilograms of hash to the United States using camper vans and other vehicles with hidden compartments, driving them to seaports and shipping them back home. According to documents uncovered by Clarke, a Brotherhood vehicle seized at Oregon customs contained 600 kilos of hash.

In 1970, a Brotherhood member named Bobby Andrist developed a method of making "honey oil," by refining Afghan hashish into a more potent, gooey, viscous, translucent, sticky substance that shone like amber. Liters

> "**The simplest words, the most trivial ideas, assume a strange new guise; you are actually astonished at having hitherto found them so simple. . . . How mysteriously comical are the feelings of a man who revels in incomprehensible mirth at the expense of anyone not in the same situation as himself!**"
>
> CHARLES BAUDELAIRE, ON SMOKING HASH

of honey oil were selling in the States for up to ten grand, until an illicit hash oil factory operated by Andrist exploded near Kabul, tipping off the first agent from the Bureau of Narcotics and Dangerous Drugs that something might be happening. Andrist and other Brotherhood members were jailed in 1972, but the smuggling of hash continued.

Head to one of Amsterdam's fine coffeeshops even today, and you can still sample a wide selection of hash from exotic locales made in the traditional fashion, under names like Manali Cream, Rif Cream, and Rifman Malika. Like fine wines, each has a *terroir* all its own, due to the soil, the weather, and sundry other factors that affected the growth of the plants and their processing into hash.

In his 2010 article "Hash Quest: Morocco" our adventurous editor Nico Escondido embedded himself with some Moroccan hash-makers, offering a comprehensive report on their ancient methods of cultivating cannabis and making hash. Falling in with a group of younger hash-makers, he learned that their methods differed very little from those of their grandfathers.

THE "GATEWAY DRUG" THEORY

A huge majority of mass murderers have eaten a carrot at least once in their lives, so therefore something about carrots must cause people to end up cold-blooded killers, right? Wrong, of course, and there's literally no more scientific basis behind the supposed "gateway theory," which says marijuana use leads to harder drugs. But why believe *High* *Times*, when the Institute of Medicine of the National Academy of Sciences did an extensive study of the subject in 1999, and decided that the whole theory's a bunch of hooey? They concluded, "there is no conclusive evidence that the drug effects of marijuana are causally linked to the subsequent abuse of other illicit drugs."

"The group set off from the house and began a short ascent up a small road that had water trickling down," Nico reports. "Soon irrigation equipment came into view, and pipes running from various wells could be seen. As we followed the water lines, the pungent aroma of marijuana smacked us in the face, until suddenly we were standing in a moonlit field of ganja stretching as far as my eyes could see. It was truly a magnificent sight to behold. As I looked around at the men on the edges of the fields holding torches, I realized how this tradition had been going on for centuries: the ritual of growing cannabis and turning it into hash high up in the mountains, and the continued pilgrimage of those like us who came seeking the goods of enlightenment."

HASH TECH 2.0

As a young woman, Mila Jansen traveled the Hippie Trail, learning everything she could about how to make hash along the way. She lived in different parts of the Himalayas from 1968 until the 1980s. Then, after many years in India, Mila returned to her home in Amsterdam and put her knowledge to work, growing plants for coffeeshops, making hash, and even cloning a rare California import known as Orange Bud.

In 1994, Mila had an epiphany, one she later described to *High Times* editor Jen Bernstein during a 2013 interview: "One night while doing the laundry and watching these clothes in the dryer, waffling around, I realized that's what we were doing with dry cannabis [to make hash], waffling it around. And I came up with the idea: We needed to get an old clothes dryer! We wrapped a screen around the drum, took away the heating, put the leftover leaf material in, and lo and behold—the kief collected at the bottom of the machine. I had invented the Pollinator!"

A revolution in hash-making technology, the Pollinator as it would later be manufactured contains a removable drum to be filled with leaf and trim. Several horizontal rods are added to increase the tumbling effect. The drum is then closed, placed back inside the machine, and spun, separating the kief from the plant material. The kief is then collected and pressed into hash.

Mila followed up this dry extraction technique with another invention called the Ice-O-Lator, which introduced to the world a simple but ingenious technique for making ice water hash. Basically, a large, porous bag containing cannabis buds, leaves, or trim is agitated in a barrel along with ice water. The cold ice causes the resin glands to break off and separate from the vegetative material, and the water is then filtered through a series of bags with small pores in the bottom, working from the largest pores to smallest in order to isolate increasing finer grades of hashish. The resin glands, also called crystals, are collected in the bottom of these bags after the water drains away, and the wet mass is next dried and cured before being marketed as "Bubble," so-called because of the way it bubbled and oozed while being heated and smoked.

Bubble, also known as ice hash or water hash, became incredibly popular through the late 1990s and 2000s, and a variety of devices designed to manufacture it entered the marketplace, many imitating Mila's inventions.

Mila followed up the Ice-O-Lator system with the Bubbleator, a small washing-machine-like piece of equipment that is specially designed for making ice water hash quickly and easily. Fans of ice water extraction praise the efficiency, safety, and potency of these methods, and top-quality bubble hash can easily approach 60 to 80 percent THC. About her inventions, Mila remarks, "We used to say, 'Trash to Stash,' since [the machines] make something wonderful out of what people throw away (trim) . . . The Ice-O-Lator hash is so very pure, I feel certain it will find its place in medicinal cannabis."

The Ice-O-Lator method of extracting trichomes led to a renaissance in domestic Dutch hash production (also known as "Nederhash") and Mila's system proved so influential that the term "Ice-O-Lator" became shorthand for really good hash. The differences in potency, texture, and flavor between this new domestic hash and the traditional imports led to the creation of two separate hash categories at the fourteenth annual Cannabis Cup in 2001, with Barney's Breakfast Bar, a famous coffeeshop, taking first place that year for an extraction of Sweet Tooth.

BHO

Butane Hash Oil (BHO), also known as honey oil, has been around since the 1970s. It just hasn't been widely available until fairly recently. Back then, the combination of the DEA cracking down on marijuana smuggling and North Americans learning how to grow top-notch pot led to the supply of such concentrates largely drying up. Occasionally honey oil could be found at a Grateful Dead parking lot or Rainbow Gathering, but because it was extremely sticky, it proved difficult for the average stoner to store, handle, or smoke. It would generally be dripped on top of bowls of buds, or smeared onto a rolling paper, always used sparingly due its expense and rarity.

Today, however, BHO and other chemical solvent-based extractions are all the rage, due to the instantaneous, face-smacking strength of the high. The rise of BHO has been possible through two developments: the wholesale price for outdoor cannabis fell precipitously, and stoners invented better ways to handle and smoke these viscous, sticky concentrates.

Starting in 2008, California outdoor pot prices began to plummet as increasing numbers of growers moved in from out of state to set up shop—a trend that only escalated following a 2009 U.S. Justice Department memo advising federal law enforcement not to prioritize prosecuting medical marijuana growers in compliance with state laws.

As a result, many longtime cultivators increased the size of their gardens, and many more wannabe hustlers flocked to the Emerald Triangle. Mediocre outdoor "turkey bag" pot harvested too early, cured poorly, and sold hastily flooded the market. As early as May 2010, *High Times* reported a pound of California outdoor selling for as low as eight hundred dollars, and by March 2011, our cover proclaimed "Pot Prices Plummet."

High Times editor Dan Skye has been reporting "from the field" for many seasons, and he's seen the change in the marketplace firsthand.

"Twenty-five years ago, growers could count on getting $5,000 or more per pound," Skye writes, "But with the introduction of liberal medical-marijuana laws and the influx of thousands of new growers arriving to take financial advantage, the California cannabis industry is getting schooled on the laws of supply and demand. Even top growers—those with reputations for high-quality pot earned over years of growing—have seen their prices fall below $2,500 per pound. Often, they'll settle for $2,000. New growers without connections can expect half of that—or even less."

The squeeze placed on outdoor growers by increasing competition and a market flooded with mediocre herb led many to consider "value-added products," like hash or honey oil. Ironically, market forces similar to those that led the Brotherhood of Eternal Love to refine cheap Afghan hashish down to BHO in the 1970s led California farmers to do the same, since the more potent, condensed, and portable your clandestine product is, the easier it is to smuggle to places where it's worth much more. And so farmers sitting on twenty-five pounds of outdoor pot that might fetch five hundred dollars a pound began converting their harvest into BHO, supplying a new demand for a highly potent product that can retail for up to sixty dollars per gram.

Around the same time, new inventions made it much easier to enjoy these oily extracts. The 2009 Cannabis Cup winner for Best Product was an item called the Vapor Swing, a titanium skillet that twists onto a special attachment for a typical bong. You use a Vapor Swing by dripping small "dabs" of concentrate onto the red-hot skillet, where it vaporizes and can be inhaled through the glass tube. Another innovative product called the Essential VAAAPP EV100 Portable Vaporizer also became very popular throughout 2010, since this small hand-held unit allowed for easy vaporization of essential oils, including cannabis concentrates. And so a combination of economic forces and new technology enabled a "perfect storm" to blow into town and change cannabis culture forever.

As *High Times* editor Bobby Black learned in his ongoing series of investigations into this new phenomenon, concentrate culture comes with new gear, fresh lingo, and mind-boggling highs.

"*High Times*' first official encounter with BHO was in June 2010 at our inaugural Medical Cannabis Cup in San Francisco, when three BHOs were entered into the Hash category. By the time our next Medical Cup rolled into Denver in April 2011, BHOs had become so prevalent that we had to change the name of the category to the Concentrate Cup. At our second annual San Fran Medical Cup in June 2011, eleven of the entries in the category were extracts rather than traditional hashes." A trend that continued, with a whopping thirty-five solvent-based extractions entered into the first fully legal U.S. Cannabis Cup in Denver on April 20, 2013, and a record-breaking sixty entries taken in San Bernardino in February 2014.

What makes these extractions different from traditional hash is the use of petroleum-based solvents like butane, propane, or naptha to strip THC and other cannabinoids away from the vegetative matter. Black explains:

"This method involves shooting a highly pressurized gaseous solvent (such as oxygen, nitrogen, carbon dioxide or, most commonly, butane) through the plant material (a process often referred to as "blasting"), then purging away the remaining solvent and scraping up what's left behind. This moist, gooey residue usually resembles raw honey, a resemblance responsible for its nickname: butane honey oil, or BHO."

IS BHO SAFE TO MAKE?

If you're a participant in cannabis culture, you've probably heard or read about somebody who tried to make BHO themselves at home, without proper knowledge, experience, and equipment, and ended up setting off a dangerous explosion. Butane is a highly flammable gas, and ignorant "backyard blasters" who use it improperly risk serious consequences for themselves and everyone else in the near vicinity.

That's why BHO is nicknamed "Blow Hands Off!" Indeed, such accidents have become common enough to engender a backlash, not to mention the human toll on people seriously injured or even killed in these incidents. *High Times* advises anyone interested in making BHO extracts to go to college first and get a chemistry degree, since these processes should be handled only by professionals. And whatever you do, never ever blast cans of butane indoors or stand near someone who's doing so!

"When blasting or purging the butane, the air in the surrounding area becomes permeated by the gas, which is then all too easily ignited by something as trivial as the electrical signal of a text-message alert on a cell phone," Black cautions readers. "In October 2010, a simple spark from a kitchen freezer ignited the butane in the air of a home in Oregon where people were making BHO, blowing the door clean off their refrigerator and straight through a wall. This past year, a number of explosions and serious injuries have been reported relating to butane extraction, including two people who were severely burned in their home outside Denver during a blasting accident, and another man in California who suffered burns over 90 percent of his body while attempting to make BHO in a motel room. For this reason, we at *High Times* strongly recommend that readers leave this extremely volatile and dangerous procedure to the pros."

> *High Times* advises anyone interested in making BHO extracts to go to college first and get a chemistry degree, since these processes should be handled only by professionals.

ARE DABS SAFE TO SMOKE?

Based on the findings of medical experts, it seems as if properly purged, professionally made BHO is okay to consume, but it's really too new of a phenomenon to have solid scientific evidence of its safety over a long period of use. In "To Dab or Not To Dab?" Black addressed these health concerns by providing substantial excerpts from a discussion he moderated at the Denver Medical Cannabis Cup, the panel for which included extract experts Selecta Nikka T and Daniel de Sailles, medical doctor Alan Shackelford, University of Colorado professor of biology Robert Melamede, and Denver *Westword* newspaper's pot critic William Breathes.

"Nearly everyone agrees that the only serious health risk posed by smoking BHO is the possibility of ingesting harmful contaminants that may have been infused into the concentrate during the extraction process," Black wrote, noting however that this can be a significant concern when so much of what's on the market is still made under black market conditions.

"The biggest concern is the quality of the marijuana—who's been growing it and what they used," said Dr. Melamede. "If you have contaminants (i.e., pesticides, herbicides, fungi) on your plant, that's going to come off into the extract. Then, when you evaporate the solvent, you'll actually be concentrating those things—and that's the real danger. Pesticides are typically extremely nasty in how they can affect your nervous and immune systems, so you definitely don't want to be consuming that."

As if incompetent blasters weren't enough, one must also be wary of criminals out to make a quick buck selling bogus product. "You have a whole spectrum of unscrupulous people out there who are going to do whatever to try to make money," continued Dr. Melamede. "I personally wouldn't use any cannabis product if I didn't know who produced it and/or hadn't had it properly analyzed."

One perfect example: a video that Breathes posted on his blog in which he dropped a chunk of "shatter" (brittle BHO) onto a hot nail, only to have it flame up high enough to scorch his face if he'd actually tried to inhale it. Later

> **"I personally wouldn't use any cannabis product if I didn't know who produced it and/or hadn't had it properly analyzed."**
>
> DR. ROBERT MELAMEDE, PROFESSOR OF BIOLOGY AT THE UNIVERSITY OF COLORADO

that week, Breathes had the sample tested and was shocked to learn that it contained only 10 percent cannabinoids (compared with 50 to 75 percent in most concentrates).

OIL RIGS

Sparked by rapidly growing consumer demand, the evolution of smokeware specifically intended for dabbing concentrates has progressed quickly, with these new "oil rigs" replacing the traditional bong. In "Concentrate Revolution," Bobby Black explains how it all works:

"Instead of a standard bowl, rigs have a nail—a small spike made of quartz or titanium. Using a high-powered lighter or small, hand-held blowtorch (such as a crème brûlée cooking torch), the nail is heated until glowing red. A small dab (hence the term dabbing) of concentrate is touched to the head of the nail using a glass or metal wand called a dabber. As soon as the concentrate begins to dissolve, the user draws in the smoke from the rig's mouthpiece in exactly the same way they would a bong. A brief coughing fit later, and abraca-DAB-ra—you're high!"

IDENTIFYING EXTRACTS

Based on the kind of cannabis alchemy used, extracts and concentrates can be thick and viscous, waxy, chunky, smooth, buttery, or hard like brittle candy.

"Generally speaking, a concentrate's consistency is just a result of how much moisture it contains," Black explains. "Which is why, when you leave certain extracts out in the air for a while, they begin to goo up—a process known as auto-buddering. Basically, by manipulating the extract in different ways (temperature, moisture, pressure, agitation), the extract artist can produce a variety of textures to appeal to all palates and preferences."

CONCENTRATED CONTROVERSY

About ten years ago, stories began to spread through the cannabis underground of a Canadian man who was treating cancer patients with a homemade, highly concentrated marijuana medicine that he dubbed "hemp oil." Chronicled in-depth by longtime editor Steven Hager in "Rick Simpson's

KNOW YOUR BHO

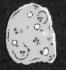

EARWAX   SAP BHO   HONEY OIL   GLASS   CRUMBLE   BUDDER

Budder — Hash oil that has been whipped. Stable and pure. More creamy than sticky.

Earwax — Slightly stickier than budder. Consistency of a paste, similar to earwax.

Glass / Shatter — Translucent, smooth amber-colored solid that "shatters" when you break off a dab.

Honey Oil — Gooey, unprocessed concentrate with the consistency of thick, sticky liquid.

Raw / Crumble — A puffed, aerated consistency like a cheese doodle. Crumbles into sand when handled.

Snap / Sap — Translucent with a consistency like taffy that "snaps" when you pull off a dab.

Hemp-Oil Medicine," the "cannabis cures cancer" claims of this iconoclast generated much excitement, amid great controversy.

After an industrial accident in 1997, Simpson was plagued by a debilitating brain injury that caused constant, loud ringing in his ears. In 2001, after watching a television documentary about the healing potential of medical marijuana, he decided to try it, and quickly found that pot helped control his pain and reduce his need for an intense regimen of prescription pharmaceuticals. Months later, Simpson's doctor informed him that they had tried every possible treatment and nothing had worked, so Rick was on his own. He decided to stop taking pharmaceuticals and start eating cannabis oil exclusively.

"I didn't really believe the hemp oil could bring me back the way it did," Simpson recalls. "But once the system gave up on me, I just continued making oil and taking it on a regular basis. The ringing was still there, but now I could live with it. Within a few months, people saw the difference. The oil controlled the pain, my blood pressure, and it allowed me to sleep. I lost weight and looked twenty years younger."

WHAT IS RSO?

Rick Simpson uses "Hemp Oil" as the term for his formula, but it shouldn't be confused with the non-psychoactive hemp seed oil you can purchase at the health food store. Most cannabis activists use the abbreviation "RSO" for Rick Simpson Oil, which has become the preferred shorthand for concentrated, edible cannabis oil, although the term "Phoenix Tears" is also used. RSO is produced in a fashion similar to BHO, using naptha, alcohol, or ether as a solvent. The resulting thick goo is purged of solvent before being dispensed through a syringe dropper so the patient can measure precise, small doses, which are ingested, not inhaled.

Simpson went on to use his concentrated cannabis oil as a topical treatment for skin cancer and weeping psoriasis. He also administered it internally to cancer patients, and based on their success resolved to freely give his medicine away to anyone in need. Which he did, until The Royal Canadian Mounted Police raided his property and seized his cannabis plants in 2003, and then again in 2005 and 2009—finally bringing an end to Simpson's generosity and forcing him into political exile in Europe.

DOES RSO ACTUALLY WORK?

Although Simpson and his followers breathlessly promote the cancer-curing potential of concentrated cannabis oil, others in the medical marijuana community urge caution. So far, largely because of the NIDA blockade on cannabis research in the United States, no solid scientific evidence backs up such claims, and although we know that cannabinoids have anti-tumor properties, many worry that touting RSO as a miraculous cure-all will give false hope to cancer patients desperately seeking to survive. Especially worrisome is the belief amongst some RSO activists that chemotherapy will counteract the healing benefits of the oil, leading patients to eschew traditional therapies.

In response to Hager's "Rick Simpson's Hemp-Oil Medicine" article, Dr. Lester Grinspoon, MD published an op-ed entitled "Medical Marijuana: A Note of Caution" in early 2010, urging activists to take a more measured approach. Dr. Grinspoon, a highly respected cannabis researcher and associate professor emeritus of psychiatry at Harvard Medical School, noted that, "Simpson, who does not have a medical or scientific education (he dropped out of school in ninth grade), apparently does not require that a candidate for his treatment have an established diagnosis of a specific type of cancer, usually achieved through biopsy, gross and histopathological examinations, radiologic and clinical laboratory evidence. He apparently accepts the word of his 'patients.' Furthermore, after he has given the course of 'hemp oil,' there is apparently no clinical or laboratory follow-up; he apparently accepts the 'patients'' belief that they have been cured."

"MILAGRO" OIL AND THE NEED FOR FURTHER STUDY

Valerie Corral at the Wo/Men's Alliance for Medical Marijuana (wamm.org) has developed a concentrated cannabis oil she calls "Milagro," which uses 190-proof ethanol alcohol to concentrate the cannabinoids. In a series of columns written for *High Times Medical Marijuana* magazine, she chronicled the experiences of several of her patients who were pursuing traditional therapies as well as cannabis oil, writing, "Most recently, WAMM has been investigating the efficacy of ingesting über-doses of high-grade, organic cannabis-oil extract in the treatment of various types of cancer. To that end, we've created a new product, Milagro Oil Extract, which in laboratory tests averaged 65 percent THC, 3.5 percent CBD and 1.5 percent CBN. Cancer patients, who must first familiarize their oncologists with their use, slowly increase their dosage until they are ingesting one gram each day, with the goal of consuming a total of 60 grams within a ninety-day period."

Addressing the complicated issue of concentrated cannabis oil as a possible cure for cancer, Clint Werner, author of *Marijuana: Gateway to Health*, writes, "The problem with talking about a 'cure' for cancer, however, is that cancer is a collective term for a variety of different disease processes that share certain common traits. For example, the development and progression of lung cancer is quite different from that of lymphoma, so while we might find that cannabis oil is effective for treating certain brain tumors, it could be ineffective for treating blood cancers."

In order for anyone to prove that Rick Simpson's homemade medicine—or any concentrated cannabis product—can cure cancer, we need to first change the draconian laws that block research and then unleash teams of scientists and doctors to study the reasons behind the anecdotal evidence of cannabis' healing benefits. Only with such scientific inquiry can the true potential of cannabis be harnessed for the benefit of all.

THE FUTURE OF CANNABIS

Despite the potential danger of producing dabs and the related PR problem of how they appear to the public, it seems that chemical solvent-derived cannabis concentrates are here to stay. These waxes and budders provide instant medicinal relief, evaporating pain immediately with pure doses of cannabinoids. Patients with Alzheimer's or cancer may find it much easier to sip a few hits from a vapor pen instead of puffing down an entire joint.

Advocates for "dab life" look forward to the widespread introduction of "e-Nails," electronic nails that heat to a precise temperature and eliminate the need for blowtorches. Colorado has put forth rigorous safety standards for production of concentrates, and mandates lab testing for any product sold in a retail store or dispensary. Together, innovation and regulation will tame the wild world of dabbing, and the public will become more accepting once educated about the benefits of concentrated cannabis.

As Bobby Black opines in his 2013 piece "Generation Dab," this latest development in the evolution of cannabis culture just might change everything: "Dabbing isn't a fad—it's a paradigm shift, and rejecting it won't make it go away. . . . To many in this up-and-coming generation of young stoners, smoking 'flowers' (as weed is now referred to) is fast becoming passé—a quaint custom practiced by hippies, lightweights, and the socio-geographically disadvantaged. . . . As word of this new way of getting stoned continues to spread and the demand for BHO grows, the market begins to respond: One-hitters are replaced by vapor pens, butane is bought in bulk, and sales of crème brûlée torches skyrocket. . . . As the focus of pot nerds everywhere slowly shifts from botany to chemistry, so shifts the spotlight from growers to the modern-day alchemists known as extract artists, who can transform a pile of leftover leaf into taffy-esque, translucent gold."

CONCENTRATES GLOSSARY

✦ ✦ ✦ ✦ ✦ ✦ ✦ ✦ ✦ ✦ ✦ ✦

**Bell
(a.k.a. Curve)** A bell-shaped glass headpiece that attaches to the stem of a standard water pipe used for smoking concentrates (see also Slide).

BHO Butane hash oil, also referred to as butane honey oil. A concentrate made by shooting butane gas through cannabis, then "purging" out the butane.

Blasting Making BHO (as in "he's blasting some flowers tomorrow").

Bubble A type of hash that bubbles up when you smoke it.

Budder-faced Getting really high on cannabis budder (i.e., "getting budder-faced").

Concentrate Any form of cannabinoid extracted from cannabis-plant material (e.g., hash, wax, tincture).

Dab A hit of extract loaded onto a wand or pick to be smoked on a rig.

Dabber A glass utensil used for smoking concentrates (see also Wand).

Dabbing Smoking a concentrate from a nail, swing, or shovel.

Dish A small, glass, ashtray-like container used to hold concentrates; usually including an indentation to rest a dabber.

**Dome
(a.k.a. Globe)** The bowl-like collar/glass cap placed over the hot nail on an oil rig to help contain the smoke and prevent injury.

Earl Slang for BHO ("oil").

Extraction Any method by which the THC and/or other cannabinoids are removed from the plant matter via a solvent.

Goo Any sticky, oozy concentrate.

Glob An especially large dab.

Hash oil A sticky, moist concentrate that has the consistency of oil.

Honeybud Cannabis buds that have been infused with BHO.

Hot-knifing A method of smoking concentrates that entails heating up the edge of a knife and then dabbing the concentrate onto it.

Ice hash (a.k.a. "water hash") A concentrate made using ice-water extraction methods (see also bubble, melt).

ISO hash (a.k.a. "QWISO," for "quick-wash ISO") A concentrate made by soaking cannabis in isopropyl alcohol as a solvent.

Kief   A dry, solvent-less, powdered concentrate derived from sieving cannabis over a fine mesh.

Melt   A very pure hash that melts fully when smoked and leaves no residue.

Nail   A spike used in place of a bowl to smoke concentrates; usually made of glass, quartz, or titanium (see iron).

Oil rig (or just "rig")   A bong designed specifically to smoke concentrates by replacing the bowl with a nail and dome.

Paddles   Long, thin glass sticks with rounded edges used to smoke concentrates by heating up and pressing together.

Purge   The act of drawing out any solvents from your concentrate (usually by whipping with low heat or by vacuum leaching).

Reclaim   The excess oil that builds up inside a rig or shovel, which can be "reclaimed" by gently heating the glass with the torch and pouring it out.

Shatter   A form of BHO that shatters when you try to scrape it up from the dish.

Shovel   A hollow paddle that can be smoked from; a paddle/bowl hybrid.

Skillet   A small metal plate used for dabbing.

Slide   A glass bowl that fits a standard water pipe that's specifically designed for smoking concentrates.

Solvent   A medium used to extract cannabinoids from plant matter (e.g., butane, ethanol, alcohol, oxygen).

Swing   A metallic plate clipped to a bong or rig and used to smoke concentrates.

Tincture   An ingestible extraction made by soaking plant matter in an edible solvent such as agave, drinking alcohol, or vegetable glycerin.

Torch   A small blowtorch (usually a handheld crème brûlée torch or propane canister) used to heat a nail or skillet for smoking concentrates.

Torching   Smoking concentrates using a torch.

Tube   A rig or bong.

Wand (a.k.a. "dropper," "dabber") A long glass tool used to scrape up and apply concentrates to a heated surface for smoking.

7:10   The unofficial time to do dabs ("OIL" spelled upside down).

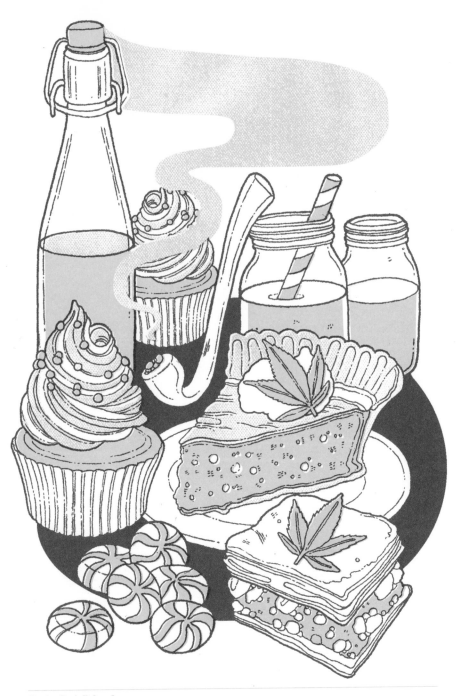

Magically delicious!

Eating Cannabis

MAGICALLY DELICIOUS

Whether you're seeking a relaxing buzz without having to inhale, long-term pain relief without dangerous pharmaceutical drugs, or a safe, effective sleep aid that leaves you feeling refreshed and rejuvenated the next day, it's high time to try a cannabis-infused edible. Just make sure you know how much THC you're ingesting, and keep in mind that eating marijuana typically gets you significantly higher than smoking the same amount.

In fact, many hard-core stoners actually swear off pot food for this reason, usually based on an unpleasant experience that resulted from biting off more herb than they could chew. While such overdoses will never prove serious or life-threatening, they can certainly make you feel highly uncomfortable for a few hours. But the good news is that in medical and recreational marijuana states, retailers now carry a wide variety of cannabis edibles—like Bhang Chocolates, Day Dreamers, Incredible Edibles, and Toffee Turtles—all of which are lab tested to provide their exact potency, so you can accurately ingest an agreeable dose every time. And Colorado requires lab testing for all edibles, while at time of writing the situation is in flux elsewhere.

> **"It makes me feel the way I need to feel."**
>
> SNOOP DOGG

COMMERCIAL CANNABIS KITCHENS

Tripp Keber, managing director of Dixie Elixirs in Colorado, predicts that the overall medical marijuana industry will be a nine billion dollar business by 2016, with edibles and other infused products providing up to 25 percent of those sales. Many small "mom and pop" companies continue to compete in this segment, even as larger players begin to establish themselves as market leaders. The industry is also pushing for improved safety standards and best practices. Dixie Elixirs, for example, developed labeling that meets FDA requirements, as well as an operating procedure that meets food safety guidelines under its Hazard Analysis and Critical Control Points (HACCP) plan.

In Colorado, state regulators enforce strict requirements for cannabis-infused foods under the direction of the Marijuana Enforcement Division, including lab testing and clear dosage information. The San Francisco Department of Health's most recent Medical Cannabis Dispensary Regulations ban items requiring refrigeration, set guidelines for a sanitary workplace, and outline acceptable packaging and labeling for cannabis-infused food items.

As the marijuana law reform movement progresses and more states legalize cannabis, this type of regulation will become the norm in the edibles industry, including mandated tamper-proof packaging, branding that doesn't appeal to children (no cartoon characters!), restrictions on advertising, health inspections of infused product facilities, and standardization of dosage levels, labeling requirements, and operating procedures. Until this fully-legal future becomes reality, however, consumers must educate themselves about how to choose the best cannabis-infused products for their needs—including the option of making them yourself at home.

KNOW YOUR DOSE

It's generally a good idea to either avoid edibles of unknown potency, or approach them with caution, since you can always eat more, but can't eat less once it's in your stomach. For purchased edibles, you ideally should be able to understand how many milligrams of THC you're going to ingest based on a clear, lab-test-confirmed label. Labels that do not offer THC info, but make promises like "double-strength" or "2X dosage" unfortunately don't really mean anything unless you know what's being doubled.

When making foods at home, a good rule of thumb is to include .5 grams of cannabis for each serving, so if your recipe yields twelve brownies, start by infusing 3 grams of ground cannabis into the amount of oil that the recipe calls for (assuming that a person will eat two brownies).

Before eating cannabis-infused food for the first time, carefully consider your personal level of experience with ganja inhalation—if any—because heavy tokers who are well accustomed to marijuana's psychoactivity will far more easily adjust to the effects of edibles than those who have a hard time handling their smoke. So be honest: Are you a one-hit-and-quit smoker or can you puff tough all night long?

For cannabis-naive folks who have never used the healing weed previously, that means starting with a very low dose of 5 milligrams of THC and working your way up slowly. Heavy smokers can start with 15 to 20 milligrams, but should keep in mind that even veteran bong rippers can sometimes be unpleasantly surprised by the strength and duration of an edibles high, which due to the way the body absorbs the THC can be much more intense than through inhalation in the lungs.

> If you are eating homemade edibles of an unknown origin—or a purchased item without THC content information—always start with a very small piece and wait at least ninety minutes before consuming more.

BUYING EDIBLES

When selecting a cannabis-infused product from the shelves of a medical marijuana dispensary or state-legal retail outlet, it's easy to be overwhelmed by the sheer variety of what's available.

At *High Times*, as part of our Cannabis Cup competitions, we evaluate hundreds of marijuana-infused foods each year, from savory dips, salad dressings, and sauces to sugary treats such as gummy bears and ice cream to healthy options like granola bars and fruit smoothies. Here are some tips for choosing the edible that's right for you:

- **Look for a product that offers an appropriate dose of THC at a satisfying portion size.** For example, a sweet tooth seeking a low dose wouldn't be happy with a tiny truffle containing 200 milligrams of THC, since that would require using a razor blade to slice off a preferred dose of 20 mg.

Nor do those trying to quell chronic neuropathic pain want to eat two slices of cheesecake every time they need relief. Pain patients who consume edibles regularly and may need 100 mg of THC per day (or more) should definitely seek out healthier options, including well-balanced, nutritious recipes to make at home.

- **Look for professional tamper-proof packaging and labeling.** This should include an ingredients list, allergy information, appropriate warnings that the item contains cannabis, dosage advice, and a 1-800 number or website that allows customers to contact the company directly with any questions or concerns. Most importantly, packaging should include lab test information that details the amount of THC and CBD in milligrams per serving, plus the amount of servings in a package. For example, a chocolate bar containing 180 total milligrams of THC can have that dose spread across six separate sections of 30 mg each.

- **Be sure the edible is clearly labeled as containing cannabis!** An obvious pot leaf on the package or very large and legible type should make that abundantly clear, to prevent accidental ingestion by a roommate, family member, babysitter, neighbor, houseguest, or anyone else who might be raiding your refrigerator. And if you have children or pets in the house, always keep edibles out of sight in a locked cabinet.

- **Consider your needs.** Choose an edible that fits into your lifestyle. If you're looking for daily pain relief, try high-dose cannabis capsules. For occasional relaxation, try a low-dose chocolate. Stock up on cannabis-infused olive oils that can be sprinkled onto a salad for quick relief.

- **Think strain-specific.** If you need daytime pain relief, use an edible that specifies *sativa* strains were used. For help sleeping, seek out indica-specific edibles.

- **Always ask your budtender for any recommendations.** A knowledgeable salesperson can help you find the edible that's right for your needs. Make sure the brand of edibles you choose has an established relationship with your dispensary.

- **Read reviews.** Especially after a *High Times* Cannabis Cup! We always rate the top ten edibles from California, Colorado, and Washington State, and you can discover which products are on the cutting edge.

EAT RIGHT!

Weight, metabolism, and many other factors can make a significant difference in how an edible affects you. For faster results, consume products on an empty stomach, since a large meal will slow down your digestion and cause the effects of the cannabis to be delayed by a few hours. (Eating a 20-milligram THC brownie on an empty stomach versus consuming it after a huge holiday meal will result in distinctly varying outcomes as far as the intensity and duration of the high.) People with fast metabolisms may feel noticeable effects from even small doses of cannabis, so if you are an athlete, start with small amounts of infused foods.

Note that while smoked or vaporized cannabis is directly absorbed through the lungs and therefore begins to reach the brain within seconds—making it easy to stop smoking once the desired effect has been reached—when you eat cannabis, the liver actually converts the plant's THC into an even more psychoactive substance known as 11-hydroxy THC. This explains why the euphoria and body stone felt after eating edibles can be so intense. (And it is—once again—why you should always wait an hour or more after ingesting a small dose of cannabis before consuming any more.)

While this may sound like common sense, overdosing on THC treats due to impatience for the effects to start is actually one of the most common mistakes people make. It typically goes down something like this: After a meal, someone eats a pot brownie, and when they haven't felt it kick in after just forty-five minutes, they decide to eat another, resulting in an overwhelming wave of psychoactivity in about two hours, when the first and second doses begin to overlap. Overdosing on edibles can be a very unpleasant experience. But if it happens to you, do not panic. It's impossible to ingest a lethal dose of THC, so while eating too much herb can be scary, just keep taking deep breaths, and after a few hours you will drift off to sleep. There's certainly no reason to freak out and visit an emergency room, even if it feels like your "soul will separate from your physical being" (as has been reported).

After eating too much THC, you may sleep for as long as twelve to twenty-four hours, depending on how overboard you went, and upon waking, you might still feel groggy for a day or so. Even when ingesting small amounts of cannabinoids, be sure to allow for a restful night of "super sleep," and get a full eight hours of it. Then, the next morning, you'll awake feeling deeply rested, ready to take on the day with renewed vigor.

HOW TO READ A LABEL

- Activated cannabinoids should be listed in milligrams, e.g.: 25mg of THC, 15mg of CBD, 1mg of CBN.
- Packaging should have prominent pot leaf and a clear "Contains Cannabis" warning and "Keep Out of Reach of Children and Animals."
- Look for a nutritional information chart, ingredients list, and any allergy warnings.
- Look for dosage advice, e.g.: "Eat one half of this product and wait one hour before consuming more." Product should not advise eating more than 25mg of THC in one serving.
- Does package list a website or 1-800 number for more information or questions?
- Packaging should be tamper-proof and hygienic.
- Labelling should note whether cannabis was infused into butter or oil. If a solvent-based extraction was used to infuse product with cannabinoids, the package should say what type of solvent was used.
- Does the packaging note specific strain information, e.g.: Was edible made with *indica* or *sativa*? What strain, or blend, specifically?

COOKING WITH GRASS

Many people, even those with access to store-bought edibles, prefer to prepare their own marijuana-infused foods, so they can tailor the recipe to match their personal tastes and dosage requirements. Cooking with cannabis at home can also be lots of fun, provided you have basic kitchen equipment and the ability to follow a recipe.

So here are the basic steps for making cannabis-infused oils and butters that can be used in a variety of recipes, from fresh fruit salads to flaky piecrusts. With these pantry staples, only your imagination is the limit when it comes to THC-infused foods. And if you happen to grow your own cannabis, that's even better, because you will be able to select your strains and maintain a consistent supply of the most important ingredient!

HELP! I'm TOO HIGH and FREAKING OUT!

- Don't panic. You're going to be fine.
- Retreat to a safe place to lie down, dim the lights, and breathe deeply.
- Drink plenty of fluids and eat non-pot food.
- Distract yourself by listening to your favorite music or watching a movie.
- You'll probably drift off to sleep. Let yourself. The effects will pass with time and you'll feel better soon.
- Keep in mind that it is **humanly impossible to fatally overdose on cannabis,** even if you've just eaten an entire birthday cake frosted with cannabis buttercream. It's estimated that the amount of THC required to cause a fatal overdose would be 4,000,000 milligrams, or about nine pounds of pure hashish—and you definitely didn't eat nearly that much or you wouldn't be able to read this sentence.

HOMEMADE HIGH RULES OF THUMB

🌿 🌿 🌿 🌿 🌿 🌿 🌿 🌿 🌿 🌿

When making foods at home, a good rule of thumb is to include .5 grams of cannabis for each serving, so if your recipe yields 12 brownies, start by infusing 3 grams of ground cannabis into the amount of oil that the recipe calls for (assuming a serving is two brownies). If you are eating homemade edibles of an unknown origin—or a purchased item without THC content information—always start with a very small piece and wait at least ninety minutes before consuming more.

SELECTING CANNABIS FOR COOKING

If you don't grow your own, be sure to source your herb from a trusted dispensary or provider. Full-service retailers will even sell trimmed off parts of their crops to customers—an excellent option to help keep your pot food affordable. Better known as "trim," these are the small "sugar leaves" that grow close to the buds and must be removed with scissors prior to smoking. Coated in resin glands—called trichomes—that contain the medicinal and psychoactive cannabinoids that get you high, they make a great "cooking stock." The larger fan leaves that grow between buds contain much lower levels of THC, and a lot more chlorophyll (which has an unpleasant "grassy" taste). So for best results, stick to sugar leaves, about two ounces for every pound of butter or oil you infuse.

A slightly higher-end option is to step up from trim to using lesser-quality buds for edibles, including so-called "popcorn nugs" that are so small they're not worth trimming, and the buds from the lower branches of the plant that don't reach full potency. Combining small buds with trim or powdery "shake" from the bottom of bags or jars is another excellent way to get ingredients for cannabis cookery without breaking the bank. When using buds or shake, aim for about an ounce per pound of butter or oil.

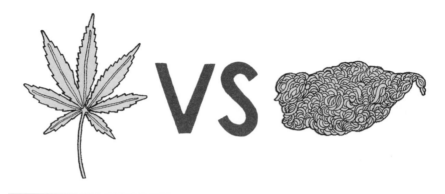

Sugar leaves and popcorn nugs are great for cooking.

Many commercial cannabis kitchens prefer to use kief—a golden powder made almost entirely of collected resin glands—or hashish, a concentration of these same resin glands that's compressed into a solid. Additional methods of making hash include solventless extraction using ice water to create bubble hash (see page 110), or by using solvents like butane or hexane to create honey oil, budder, or shatter (see page 111). Most solvent-based extractions are considered too costly and valuable to cook with, but some hash oil does find its way into commercial edibles. It's useful for making drinks, though some people feel it leaves a harsh acrid aftertaste. Coarse grades of bubble hash are excellent for cooking, imparting a rich, earthy flavor, high potency, and a somewhat more affordable price tag. Using hash or kief means avoiding the grassy taste of trim, and just 5 to 10 grams of hash will properly infuse a pound of butter or oil.

FUNDAMENTALS OF *HIGHLY* ELEVATED FOOD

Here are simple recipes for basic infusions of cannabis into fat, with more detailed instruction for those so inclined (hello decarboxylation!). The recipes that follow will use these as foundations, and you can use them in your own recipes and cooking in a variety of methods. Creating new recipes while stoned in the kitchen can be amazing fun, and many chefs smoke pot for the sensory-boosting effects that make every meal into a sublime experience. New York restaurateur Eddie Huang told *High Times* in a 2013 interview that besides using cannabis to unwind from a busy day, he also uses it to brainstorm new dishes, saying, "I have this recipe document on Google, and

Table of Equivalents

The exact equivalents in the following tables have been rounded for convenience.

LIQUID/DRY MEASUREMENTS

US	METRIC
¼ teaspoon	1.25 milliliters
½ teaspoon	2.5 milliliters
1 teaspoon	5 milliliters
1 tablespoon (3 teaspoons)	15 milliliters
1 fluid ounce (2 tablespooons)	30 milliliters
¼ cup	60 milliliters
⅓ cup	80 milliliters
½ cup	120 milliliters
1 cup	240 milliliters
1 pint (2 cups)	480 milliliters
1 quart (4 cups, 32 ounces)	960 milliliters
1 gallon (4 quarts)	3.84 liters
1 ounce (by weight)	28 grams
1 pound	448 grams
2.2 pounds	1 kilogram

LENGTHS

US	METRIC
⅛ inch	3 millimeters
¼ inch	6 millimeters
½ inch	12 millimeters
1 inch	2.5 centimeters

OVEN TEMPERATURES

FAHRENHEIT	CELSIUS	GAS
250	120	½
275	140	1
300	150	2
325	160	3
350	180	4
375	190	5
400	200	6
425	220	7
450	230	8
475	240	9
500	260	10

anytime I'm high, I'll have it open when I'm at the crib and I just start plugging things in because I know that I'm going to get ideas . . . it's also that, when you are high, you wanna think about food. I think about food and I think about sex and that's pretty much it when I'm high."

CANNABIS INFUSION PER POUND OF BUTTER

INGREDIENT	AMOUNT
TRIM	2 ounces
BUD	1 ounce
HASH	10 grams

THC Oil

It's not necessary to use first-pressed extra-virgin or estate-bottled olive oil to make your THC oil; an affordable virgin olive oil works nicely. Of course, high-quality ingredients result in a more delicious end product, so if you plan on using your THC oil for salad dressings or to drizzle over veggies and pasta, a fruity extra-virgin olive oil will make all the difference.

MAKES 6 CUPS

6 cups olive oil or canola oil

1 ounce cannabis buds, finely ground, or 2 ounces trimmed leaf, dried and ground

1. In a double boiler, slowly heat oil on low heat for a few minutes until you begin to smell the oil's aroma. Add the ground cannabis slowly, stirring until it is fully coated before adding more cannabis. Simmer on low heat for 45 minutes, stirring occasionally.

2. Remove the mixture from heat and allow it to cool before straining. Press the plant matter with the back of a spoon to wring all the oil out of it. Compost the leafy remains and save the oil in an airtight container in the refrigerator for up to two months.

Scientific Cannabutter

Developed by Tamar Wise, the former head of science for Dixie Elixirs, this recipe for foolproof cannabis infusions fully activates THC for the most potent products possible!

MAKES 1 ½ CUP

1 ounce cannabis flowers

2 ounces Everclear alcohol

2 cups (4 sticks) unsalted butter

1. Preheat the oven to 240° F.

2. Grind the flowers down in a blender or food processor. Spread ground flowers evenly on bottom of a sheet pan and place in the middle of the oven.

3. Bake for one hour, turning the flowers once halfway through and keeping them. Remove the pan from the oven and allow to cool for 10 minutes.

4. Place the alcohol in a spray bottle and spray a fine mist of alcohol over the toasted flowers. This step helps break down the cellulose slightly, allowing for a less green infusion color. Let flowers sit for 10 to 15 minutes.

5. Meanwhile, begin melting your butter over low heat. Because we have already decarboxylated, the butter only needs to be hot enough to extract the cannabinoids.

6. Add the flowers to the butter and stir. Keep the mixture at a low, slow simmer for at least a half hour, up to a few hours, stirring occasionally. Remove from heat and let cool for at least 20 minutes. If using a slow cooker, set to low for 6 to 8 hours and stir every hour or so to prevent burning.

7. When you have finished infusing the cannabutter, remove from heat and let cool for at least 20 minutes.

8. Line a metal strainer with cheesecloth. Pour the butter mixture through the cloth and press with the back of a spoon.

9. Your cannabutter is now ready to use in recipes! Keep it in the fridge and use within two weeks.

Cannacoconut Oil

Coconut oil has many advantages over animal products. It's a saturated fat, allowing maximum absorption of cannabinoids, but it's much healthier for you than saturated animal fat. Coconut oil is definitely the best option for vegans, and those concerned about health.

MAKES 1³/₄ CUPS

1 ounce cannabis, dried, or 2 ounces trimmed leaf

One 14-ounce jar coconut oil

1. Fill a large stockpot halfway with water, and add your cannabis. Simmer over low heat, stirring occasionally, for 1 hour. Then, add your coconut oil, and return to a simmer. Remove from heat. Let the coconut oil mixture sit for two days as it slowly extracts, in a covered pot at room temperature. Then, reheat the oil, cannabis, and water mixture until the oil melts.

2. Strain the mixture, being sure to press the plant matter firmly against the side of the strainer. Refrigerate the oil and water mixture for at least 24 hours.

3. Return the next day and separate the solidified oil from the water. Pat dry with a paper towel, then melt the cannacoconut oil in a saucepan until it is liquid. Measure into glass jars for easy dosing. Baby food jars work well.

ACTIVE INGREDIENTS

According to testing done by Cannalytics, Michigan's premier cannabis analytical laboratory, about a quarter of all edibles on the market were under 50 percent activated, and almost half of the 204 products tested were under 80 percent activated. So what does "activation" mean?

You might be surprised to find out that cannabis in its raw form isn't psychoactive at all. A person could eat the fresh leaves and buds and receive little to no euphoric effects, since the living, green cannabis plant contains cannabinoids only in their acidic form. The acidic form of THC is called THCA, and lab testing can show the amount of THCA left in a baked good or food item, thus revealing how much potential THC was left inactive. In order to change THCA into THC and activate its psychoactivity, a chemical reaction must occur.

Molecules of THCA have a COOH carboxyl group of atoms attached. When the plant matter is heated or dried, the COOH carboxyl group of atoms leaves the plant matter, exiting as water and carbon dioxide. This process is known as decarboxylation, or "decarb," and how well it works is a function of time and temperature. As plants dry and buds cure, the THCA is slowly converted to THC. When cannabis is smoked, the heat of combustion causes decarboxylation to occur rapidly as we inhale. THC boils at 314°F, and CBD at 356°F, and the other cannabinoids and terpenes are activated at various temperatures.

To make potent edibles quickly: If you wish to speed up the process, you can heat the herb to 293°F for as little as seven minutes, but you must remove it from heat immediately. Too much heat for too long will cause THC to convert into CBN, which is known for its sedative qualities. To make potent edibles slowly: You can also go low and slow, and heat your cannabis in oil or butter at 176°F for an hour or more. Heating to 240°F for 45 minutes to an hour will be the most efficient way to proceed, so be sure to use a candy thermometer to check the temperature of your infusion. If you are using a Crock-Pot, consult your owner's manual since models vary, but generally the Low setting is about 200°F and the High setting is 300°F.

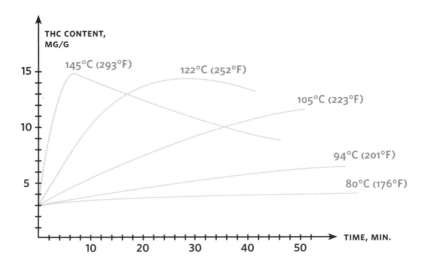

Effect of heating time and temperature on the THC content of an o-hexane marijuana extract.

TO DECARB OR NOT TO DECARB

Some stoner chefs recommend "decarbing" your plant material by toasting it in an oven before you add it to any fat-based infusion. This step can be helpful to ensure you have completely activated all of the THC in your cannabis, or if you'd like to dry out wet, fresh cannabis and remove some of the grassy taste. While this means an extra step in production, it will result in more potent edibles. You can do this by simply spreading out ground-up trimmed leaves, buds, or hash onto a baking sheet, and baking in the oven at 240° for an hour. Be sure to rotate the tray several times to avoid overheating due to any oven hot spots. You can then add oven-toasted herb directly into recipes, or quickly simmer into a fat and strain the plant material away as usual.

If you decarb your cannabis into butter or oil at 250°F for thirty minutes, then simmer it in a recipe along with other ingredients at 200°F for another thirty minutes, you should have activated almost all of the cannabinoids.

HIGH AND HEALTHY

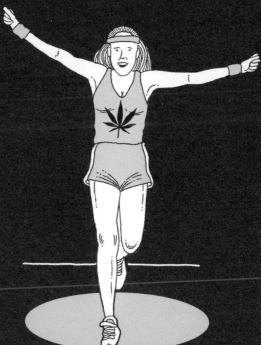

Remarkably, recent studies have shown that pot smokers are less likely to be obese than those who don't partake, even though the legendary "munchies" effect can cause a typical head to consume about 600 more calories per day than a non-user. Research completed by scientists from the University of Nebraska, the Harvard School of Public Health, and Beth Israel Deaconess Medical Center published in *The American Journal of Medicine* found that pot lovers had higher levels of HDL ("good cholesterol") and low levels of insulin, implying that cannabis somehow regulates metabolism, blood sugar levels, and insulin control.

Keep your high healthy and avoid munching down on empty calories, foods with unhealthy additives, and too much sugar. Seasoned stoners stock the house with healthy options like fresh berries, popcorn, nuts, and *sparing* amounts of (admittedly delicious) sweet-and-salty treats like chocolate-covered pretzels. Before you get baked, be sure to bake some nice oatmeal cookies, plus cut up some carrot sticks and whip up some homemade hummus, and you'll be munching happily and healthfully.

Shiva's *Sativa* Bhang

Enjoyed for thousands of years by Hindus, this spiritually inspired cannabis-infused libation is best enjoyed warm, and is traditionally drunk at the celebration of Holi, which honors Lord Shiva, a Hindu god who's known for his love of cannabis. The annual spring celebration includes an evening of bonfires and a carnival of color, where people decorate each other with brightly colored pigments and dyes. It's a day when social conventions are set aside, and things usually forbidden (such as cannabis) are indulged in. Cannabis infuses easily into the whole fat of milk, and you can use cow or goat's milk for this basic recipe.

STONES **2**

2 cups water

1 ounce cannabis (fresh leaves and flowers of a female plant preferred)

4 cups warm milk

2 tablespoons blanched, chopped almonds

⅛ teaspoon garam masala (a mixture of cloves, cinnamon, and cardamom, available at well-stocked grocery stores or Indian specialty groceries)

¼ teaspoon powdered ginger

½ to 1 teaspoon rosewater

1 cup sugar

EQUIPMENT

Cheesecloth

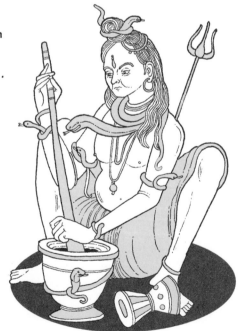

continued . . .

1. Bring the water to a rapid boil and pour into a clean teapot. Remove any seeds or twigs from the cannabis, add it to the teapot, and cover. Let this brew for about 7 minutes.

2. Strain the water and cannabis through a piece of cheesecloth (or a coffee filter), and reserve the water. Squeeze the leaves and flowers between your hands to extract any liquid that remains. Add this extract to the water and set water aside.

3. Place the leaves and flowers in a mortar and add 2 teaspoons warm milk. Slowly but firmly grind the milk and leaves together. Strain the marijuana through cheesecloth, squeezing out as much milk as you can. Repeat this process about four to five times, until you have used about ½ cup of milk. Set this milk aside.

4. By this time the cannabis will have turned into a pulpy mass. Add the almonds and another 2 teaspoons warm milk. Grind this in the mortar until a fine paste is formed. Squeeze this paste through the cheesecloth and collect the extract as before. Repeat this process a few more times until all that is left are some fibers and nut meal. Discard the residue.

5. Now combine extract with the infused milk and water you set aside previously. Add garam masala, ginger, rosewater, sugar, and remaining milk. Warm it up in a saucepan for about 3 minutes, then serve and enjoy.

Mike's Medicated Meyer Lemonade

This recipe from cannabis activist and raw foods enthusiast Chef Mike Delao features THC-infused glycerin and freshly juiced cannabis buds. Fresh leaves won't get you high, but they contain acidic cannabinoids that are great for your health! This delicious lemonade uses mild, sweet Meyer lemons, although regular lemons would work well too. Use organic veggies if available. You'll need a juicer for this recipe. If you don't have one, get one! Juicing is an excellent way to deliver important enzymes and easily absorbable vitamins into your system, allowing rejuvenation from the inside out.

STONES 2

1 ounce cannabis glycerin tincture (see Skunk Pharm Tincture, page 158)

4 Meyer lemons (or 5 regular lemons, which will yield a more tart result), peeled

3 small tangerines, peeled

3 medium-sized whole carrots, cut into chunks

2 stalks of celery, cut into chunks

1-inch piece of ginger root, peeled

3 small branches of fresh cannabis (buds or leaves)

½ cucumber, cut into chunks

EQUIPMENT

juicer

1. Thoroughly wash all your fruits and vegetables, and make sure your cannabis is free of pests and mold before you juice it. Cut the veggies into chunks that are small enough to fit easily through the juicer tube. Be sure to have a large glass or small pitcher ready to capture the juice.

2. Add the THC glycerin tincture to the bottom of the glass. When you're ready, turn on the juicer and feed lemons and tangerines through the tube first, one at a time, so their acids will blend with the glycerin. Then add carrots, celery, ginger root, and fresh cannabis, finishing with the cucumber to help flush out the machine. Stir the juice well to mix in the tincture, and skim any foam off the top. If juice tastes too "green," add another lemon. If it's too acidic, add a touch of liquid sweetener like agave nectar or honey.

3. Juice can also be saved in the fridge for a few hours, but as with most juice, it's best when fresh!

Pot Pickled Veggies

Inspired by a recipe from healthy living guru Dr. Andrew Weil, a *High Times* contributor back in his younger days, these pickles include one extra special seasoning, since the dressing contains a THC-laden olive oil. The liquid from the pickles can do double-duty as a salad dressing once the pickles have been devoured, so make sure you use every bit of that medicated oil.

This is a recipe where the cannabis should be toasted in the oven at 250°F for 30 minutes before being simmered in olive oil for another 30 minutes in order to activate all of the THC present in your cannabis. Strain the pot out of the olive oil, pressing the vegetable matter thoroughly and wringing out all the oil before discarding it. Before you start, find the jars or container that you'll use to store the pickles, and make sure the carrots and jicama are cut short enough to stand up inside.

STONES 6 TO 8

½ pound carrots, peeled and cut into thin ¾-inch sticks

½ pound string beans

1 small head cauliflower, broken into florets (about two cups)

½ raw jicama, peeled and cut into thin ¾-inch sticks

PICKLING LIQUID

2 cups water

2½ cups apple cider vinegar

¼ cup cannabis-infused olive oil (see page 136)

3 tablespoons brown sugar

1 teaspoon salt

1 tablespoon dill weed

6 cloves of garlic

¼ cup pickling spices or: 5 bay leaves, 1 tablespoon mustard seed, 1 tablespoon dill seed, and 1½ teaspoons red chili flakes

continued . . .

1. Start with a large pot and add 5 cups of water. Bring this to a boil over high heat. Prepare an ice bath in a large bowl. When the water is boiling, add the carrots first and boil for 5 minutes. Remove them with tongs or a strainer and shock them in the ice bath. Add the string beans and cook for 3 minutes, before straining and shocking in the ice water. Add the cauliflower for one minute before shocking. This step slightly cooks the vegetables and makes them more porous so the dressing can seep inside. Once the veggies are cool, strain them and drain well. Add the raw jicama.

2. To make the pickling liquid, take the ingredients and pour into a pan set over medium heat. Bring to a boil and cook for two minutes. Pour the liquid over the veggies and let them cool to room temperature. Hold your jar angled horizontally and use a chopstick to force carrots, beans and jicama into neat, upright rows, adding cauliflower here and there. Once the jars are packed, fill with dressing and refrigerate for at least two days and up to five days. In the fridge, the oil will separate and float on top of the jar. Return the jar to room temp and shake before snacking. Eat just a few pickles at a time until you get a sense of how strong the cannabis effect will be.

The "Beetnik" Burger

This veggie burger uses just a little bit of cannabis, but plenty of hemp to add extra nutrients and essential fatty acids to an already delicious patty. You could use cannabis-infused oil to fry the burgers, but a relatively small amount will be absorbed into the food and much will be wasted. Add medicated goodness with a dollop of Pot Pesto Mayo, the accompanying sauce. Using medicated sauces enables flexibility in meal planning, especially if several different people are sharing a meal.

The frozen, store-bought patties seem like cardboard compared to homemade veggie burgers like these, bursting with flavor and whole foods. This is a relatively involved recipe, with passive time to let the mixture properly set up in the fridge. You can roast the beets and other veggies ahead of time, earlier in the week. Then you can prepare the mixture in a short amount of time and have the burgers the next day. These burgers also freeze well if individually wrapped in plastic, and you can fry them up anytime! Hemp seeds can be found in well-stocked health food stores.

STONES **6** TO **8**

1 pound of red beets

½ cup brown rice

1 teaspoon olive oil (un-infused)

1 medium yellow onion, diced very fine

1 small carrot, shredded

1 celery stick, diced very fine

4 cloves garlic, minced

2 tablespoons cider vinegar

½ cup hulled hemp seeds, divided

2 crackers or a tablespoon of breadcrumbs

2 15.5-ounce cans of organic black beans

¼ cup prunes, chopped small

1 tablespoon cannabis-infused olive oil (see page 136)

½ tablespoon adobo sauce

1 chipotle chili, chopped

½ tablespoon tahini

1 tablespoon smoked paprika

2 teaspoons brown mustard

1 teaspoon cumin

½ teaspoon coriander

½ teaspoon dried thyme

1 large egg

Additional, un-infused olive oil for frying

Salt and pepper

continued . . .

TO SERVE

Goat cheese to top

6 large English muffins

Arugula

Pot Pesto Mayo
(see page 150)

1. Preheat the oven to 400°F and wrap the beets in aluminum foil. Roast for an hour. Stab the beets with a small knife; it should meet little to no resistance when the beets are done. Let the beets cool to room temperature. (This step can be done several days before you are planning to make the burgers, just save the beets in the fridge.)

2. While you are roasting the beets, bring 1 cup of water to boil in a small pot. Add a few teaspoons of salt and the rice. Reduce the heat to very low and cook the rice for 45 minutes or until all the water has been absorbed.

3. Heat a teaspoon of olive oil in a large skillet over medium heat. Add the onions, carrots and celery (this combination is referred to as mirepoix) and a little salt. Caramelize the mirepoix, stirring occasionally, and cook for 10 minutes, until the veggies are golden brown and significantly reduced in size. Add the garlic and cook for 30 seconds. Deglaze the pan by pouring in the apple cider vinegar and scraping the bottom of the pan to get all the flavor. Once the vinegar has evaporated, set the mixture aside to cool.

4. Process ¼ cup of the hemp seed and cracker or bread-crumbs in the food processor until you have a very fine meal. Transfer to a bowl and reserve for later.

5. Drain and rinse the cans of beans and add to the food processor along with the prunes. Hit the pulse button 6 to 10 times, until the beans are chopped but not too mushy. Transfer these beans to a large mixing bowl.

6. Peel the roasted beets with a peeler or edge of a spoon. Chop the beets into chunks and feed them into the food processor's grating disc, or grate with a box grater. Put the grated beets in a strainer set over the sink, and place a plate over them. Weight down the plate with a large, heavy object like a full jug of water. Press beets for at least 15 minutes.

7. Add the grated beets, cooked rice, and caramelized mirepoix to the bean mixture. Add the cannabis-infused oil, hulled hemp seeds, adobo sauce, chipotle pepper, tahini, paprika, mustard, cumin, coriander, and thyme and mix thoroughly. Add the ground hemp and bread-crumbs, plus the egg, and mix well until all ingredients are moist. Cover the mixture and refrigerate for at least four hours, or ideally overnight. This time allows the mixture to set up and the flavors to meld. Mixture will keep refrigerated for up to three days.

8. When you're ready to make the burgers, preheat the oven to 300°F and set a baking sheet on a middle rack. Scoop a ¼ cup of the mixture and form it between your palms into a flat patty about ½ thick. Heat a table-spoon of (uninfused) olive oil in a cast iron skillet or a stainless steel pan over high heat. Cook patties for a few minutes on each side, until golden brown with a nice crust. You will need to reduce the heat and add more olive oil as you go. Transfer patties to oven to keep warm as you cook the others, and add a dollop of goat cheese to melt slightly. The English muffins can be toasted for a few minutes at the same time.

9. Assemble the finished burger with toasted English muffins, goat cheese, arugula, Pot Pesto Mayo, mustard or whatever other fixings you might want. Enjoy! These burgers are lightly dosed, with just a smattering of THC, so plan on eating another burger or adding more sauce to get more medicated.

Pot Pesto Mayo

This delicious sauce has a savory, nutty, herbal flavor that blends well with cannabis. You can keep this in the fridge for up to three days, and slather it on anything—crackers, sandwiches, or pasta.

STONES **4** TO **6**

1 cup fresh basil leaves (packed down)

⅓ cup toasted walnuts

2 tablespoons of hulled hemp seeds

2 garlic cloves, minced

½ teaspoon salt

¼ teaspoon pepper

¼ cup cannabis-infused olive oil (see page 136)

¼ cup parmesan cheese, grated

¼ cup mayonnaise

1. Combine the basil, toasted walnuts, hemp seeds, garlic, salt, and pepper in the food processor and puree. Stop the machine after 30 seconds and use a rubber spatula to scrape down the sides of the bowl. Start the machine again, and as it is running, drizzle the cannabis-infused olive oil through the feeder tube. Process until it resembles a thick paste. Add the cheese and pulse a few times until it has been combined. Transfer to a container and mix the mayo in until it has been thoroughly combined. Cover tightly and refrigerate until ready to use!

Baked Sweet Potato Fries

Sweet potatoes contain complex carbohydrates and are rich in Vitamin A, beta-carotene, and antioxidants, making them a much healthier choice than white potatoes. Bake up these sweet-and-salty delicious fries as an accompaniment to the "Beetnik" Burger, and revel in the feelings of good health!

STONES **4** TO **6**

4 large sweet potatoes

1 teaspoon cornstarch

2 tablespoons cannabis-infused olive oil (see page 136)

1 teaspoon brown sugar

2 teaspoons salt

1 teaspoon pepper

2 teaspoons paprika

¼ teaspoon cayenne pepper

1. Preheat the oven to 450°F. Peel the sweet potatoes and cut into long, thin pieces about as big as a finger. Making sure all the pieces are uniform will ensure even cooking.

2. Place the cut potatoes in a plastic bag or large bowl. Add the cornstarch by sprinkling it over, then pour in the cannabis-infused olive oil, sugar, and spices and shake up the bag to coat the potatoes. If using a bowl, stir thoroughly or cover with another bowl, and holding the two bowls together, shake vigorously to coat.

3. Arrange fries in a single layer on one or two baking sheets. Don't overcrowd or the fries won't get crispy.

4. Bake for 15 minutes, then rotate the baking sheet and flip the fries over using a spatula. Bake for another 10 to 15 minutes, until the fries are crispy and the edges start to turn brown. The surface of the fries should change from shiny to a puffed-up, matte texture, and you'll know they are just about done. Enjoy!

Cannabis Coconut Mango Balls

Have you heard that eating mangoes will make the effects of pot more potent? Apparently, the terpene myrcene helps THC get to the brain faster, reportedly lengthening the high felt after smoking and increasing the euphoria. Myrcene is found in ripe mangoes (as well as cannabis), and while no scientific studies have been done to determine if this is a true effect, mangoes are so good you should be eating them anyway! Eat a fresh, very ripe mango one hour before you get high, since this gives the myrcene time to get into your bloodstream. Investigate this delicious rumor thoroughly, and pay close attention to how you feel after eating these zesty sweet treats. Perfect as a light dessert or anytime snack, these raw balls are so easy to make that they'll become a favorite in your house.

STONES **10**

3 cups shredded unsweetened coconut, plus an extra ⅓ cup for rolling

2 cups dried unsulphured mangos, soaked in water for at least 30 minutes

½ cup agave nectar

8 tablespoons cannacoconut oil (see page 138)

2 teaspoons freshly grated lemon zest

½ cup chopped almonds or macadamia nuts

1. Place all ingredients (except the ⅓ cup coconut for coating) into the food processor and pulse until well combined. Use a heaping tablespoon to measure the balls, and use your hands to roll them into a sphere shape. Roll in the shredded coconut to coat. Freeze on a parchment-covered baking sheet for 20 minutes. Store in a container in the fridge, or eat immediately! Should make about 25 balls.

Classic Cannabis Brownies

Long before California first legalized medical cannabis in 1996, Mary Jane Rathbun—better known to her many admirers as Brownie Mary—took the law into her own hands (and kitchen), personally supplying thousands of people suffering from AIDS, cancer, and other serious illnesses with her namesake medicated desserts. She also played a primary role in the campaign to pass Proposition 215, which made California the first state to allow cannabis use for medicinal purposes. Here's a classic recipe for these "magically delicious" treats.

STONES 16

1 cup all-purpose flour

¼ cup unsweetened cocoa powder

½ teaspoon baking powder

¼ teaspoon salt

3 tablespoons cannabis-infused vegetable oil (see page 136, substituting vegetable for olive oil)

5 ounces semisweet chocolate, chopped

1½ tablespoons light corn syrup

1 cup firmly packed light brown sugar

1 tablespoon applesauce

3 egg whites

2 teaspoons vanilla

1. Preheat the oven to 350°F.

2. In a small bowl, mix together the flour, cocoa powder, baking powder, and salt, and set aside.

3. Pour the THC oil and chopped chocolate into a double boiler over high heat. As the water boils in the lower pan, whisk the chocolate and oil until melted and smooth. Remove from heat and whisk in the corn syrup, brown sugar, and applesauce. Stir in the egg whites and vanilla. Beat the mixture vigorously until smooth, then stir in the flour mixture until well incorporated.

4. Grease a 9-by-13-inch baking pan. Pour the batter into the pan. Bake for 18 to 23 minutes, or until the center top is almost firm to the touch. Let cool. Enjoy.

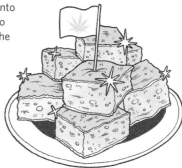

BUTTERLY LOVE

Add some culinary flair to your cannabutter by blending in spicy, sweet, savory, or floral ingredients with these recipes from *High Times Medical Marijuana* contributor Ed Murrieta.

In French kitchens, they call it *beurre composé*. In American kitchens, butter plus another ingredient—herb, spice, or nut—is known as "compound butter," our own blunt description of churned dairy blended with flavors and textures. And in medical cannabis kitchens, the most common compound butter, naturally, is cannabutter—a blending of butter and cannabis that infuses the herb's medicinal essence throughout everybody's favorite emulsion, providing a key ingredient in many edibles. But why stop there? If you can measure spices, chop nuts, melt chocolate, mince herbs, and stir a spatula, compound cannabutters are easy to make and will add true flair and flavor to your medicated treats.

In restaurants, sweet, savory, spicy, or floral compound butters are served with fresh bread. Chefs use herbed compound butters to brighten flavors and ease the acidity in wine sauces. One of my favorite steakhouses beefs up flavor with a creamy knob of pistachio-ginger butter on its grilled New York strip.

At home, you can enjoy compound cannabutters on bagels, biscuits, crepes, crackers, toast or tortillas, or atop oatmeal and pancakes. Flavor your cannabutter with orange zest, honey, and Cointreau and you'll never miss marmalade.

COMPOUND CONSIDERATIONS

Depending on the strain of medicine and the blending method you use, your compound-cannabutter flavors can range from pleasantly floral to overly herbaceous, with colors ranging from greenish-yellow to darker shades of Gumby. Choose your additions accordingly: For example, saffron vanishes in a strong cannabutter, while cinnamon survives. To get you started, check out the favorite combinations on page 156.

Chocolate-Orange Cannabutter

USE IN SMALL DOSES UNTIL YOU ARE ACCUSTOMED TO THE EFFECTS

4 ounces cannabutter
(see page 137)

1 tablespoon dark cocoa
powder

1 tablespoon finely grated
orange zest

1 tablespoon powdered
sugar

1 tablespoon finely
chopped hazelnuts
(optional)

1½ ounces dark,
bittersweet chocolate or
chocolate chips

1. Place the room-temperature cannabutter in a bowl and beat with a spatula until light and creamy; alternatively, cream the cannabutter with a hand or stand mixer. Add the cocoa powder, orange zest, powdered sugar, and hazelnuts (if desired), then mix until blended.

2. Melt the chocolate in a microwave-safe bowl on low at 20-second intervals, stirring until melted and smooth. Let it cool to the touch and then beat the chocolate into the cannabutter until smooth. Portion and store as you would any cannabutter. Serve on breads, muffins, waffles, pancakes, or crepes.

3. For a Mexican-chocolate twist, replace the orange zest with 1 teaspoon cinnamon and use almonds instead of hazelnuts.

COMPOUND FLAVORS AND TEXTURES

Ready to get compounded daily? Here are some additional flavors and textures worth exploring.

FLAVORS

- **Spicy:** cayenne chili powder, peppercorns, cinnamon, nutmeg, cardamom
- **Fruity:** purees of mango, strawberry, raspberry, or banana
- **Sweet:** chocolate, honey, molasses
- **Savory:** roasted garlic, onion, mushrooms
- **Herbal:** basil, parsley, lavender, rosemary
- **Exotic:** ginger, lemongrass (fresh, candied, or pickled)

TEXTURES

- **Nuts** (pistachios, almonds, hazelnuts—fresh or roasted)
- **Seeds** (pumpkin seeds, pine nuts, etc.—roasted and salted)
- **Coconut** (sweetened, shredded, or freshly shaved)
- **Zest** (lemon, orange, grapefruit—fresh or candied)

TINCTURES

Creating simple herbal extracts called tinctures from cannabis plants in your garden or basement is simple and easy. Well-stocked dispensaries and retail stores also carry tinctures, which are dispensed orally with a dropper. Sublingual administration allows cannabinoids to be absorbed transdermally through the numerous blood vessels under the tongue. Just let a drop of tincture sit under your tongue for a few seconds, then swish it around in your mouth. After about ten minutes, you will begin to feel the effects.

When preparing to make tincture, gather trimmed sugar leaves, plus small "popcorn" buds. Adding kief or hash will give your tincture a delicious taste, as will adding flavorful essential oils from other plants and flowers.

Alaskan King Crab *with* Tinctured Cantaloupe, Avocado Puree, *and* Cilantro Brown Butter

At hot spot bistro Cache Cache, Chef Chris Lanter caters to Aspen, Colorado's movers and shakers nightly, without ever losing sight of the upscale city's casual, countercultural roots. These days, few places offer finer dining at a higher elevation than Aspen, so it's no surprise to learn that this amazingly elegant dish appears regularly, by popular demand, on Cache Cache's menu (minus the secret ingredient, of course). To make it into a medicinal dish for patients, Chef Lanter simply infuses a cannabis tincture into the cantaloupe and viola!

STONES 4

1 pound cooked Alaskan King crab legs

2 ripe avocados

¼ pound unsalted butter

½ ripe cantaloupe, finely diced

2 ounces Skunk Pharm Tincture (see page 158)

4 tablespoons cilantro, minced

juice of 1 lemon

1. Remove crab legs from shell, cut into 3-inch chunks, and save any knuckle meat and put to side.

2. Pit avocadoes and put into food processor; add touch of salt and blend until smooth; put to side.

3. To make the Cilantro Brown Butter, chop the ¼ pound unsalted butter into eight pieces and place in pan. Cook butter over medium heat, stirring often, until foam subsides and butter solids turn light brown and smell nutty; put to side (keep warm).

4. In small mixing bowl, mix two liquid ounces of tincture with diced cantaloupe; let sit for 5 minutes.

5. To serve, spoon three tablespoons of tinctured cantaloupe onto each serving plate. Place any knuckle meat on top of tinctured cantaloupe, and one 3-inch crab chunk on top of knuckle meat. Scoop three dollops of avocado puree on each plate (next to the crab). Add cilantro and lemon juice to brown butter right before serving. Spoon over crab to taste.

6. Dine and relax!

Skunk Pharm Tincture

Developed by the researchers at Oregon's favorite cannabis school, this tincture method uses heat to activate cannabinoids, plus it's a fairly quick and easy recipe. To decarboxylate the tincture, you'll need either a fondue pot or a double boiler and candy thermometer.

USE IN SMALL DOSES UNTIL YOU ARE ACCUSTOMED TO THE EFFECTS.

14 grams trimmed leaves, or 7 grams bud and shake, or 3½ grams kief or hash

2¾ ounces vegetable glycerin

3½ cups canola oil

EQUIPMENT

Cheesecloth

Fondue pot

Candy thermometer

1. Break up any buds you might be using, but don't grind too finely, since we'll be filtering this extract later, and finely ground material makes it difficult to remove. Fill a mason jar two-thirds of the way with buds, trim, kief, or shake. Avoid using stems as they don't taste great.

2. Pour glycerin over buds, stirring with a wooden spoon until glycerin has coated all of the plant material. Top off the jar with another inch of glycerin to cover all.

3. Set the fondue pot to 200°F and fill with canola oil. Use a candy thermometer to check the temperature. Place the tincture jar in the fondue pot and stir until the glycerin mixture reaches 180°F. Turn the controls down on the fondue pot to maintain 180°F for thirty minutes, stirring regularly.

4. Remove the tincture from the fondue pot and allow it to cool to room temperature. Once the jar is cool, place it back into the fondue pot again and stir continuously until the glycerin reaches 180°F again for about five minutes. Remove and allow the jar to cool until it reaches room temperature. Repeat Step 4 at least three times and up to five times, since the repeated heating and cooling will increase the potency of your tincture.

5. After the final round of heating, remove the jar and pour the still-hot glycerin mixture through a fine metal strainer lined with cheesecloth. Drain the tincture though this filter and capture the finished product in a large glass bowl. Once cooled, squeeze the cheesecloth tightly to force more glycerin through. Discard the plant material. Store it in opaque dropper bottles in the refrigerator. Your finished tincture will last for six months in a cool dry place.

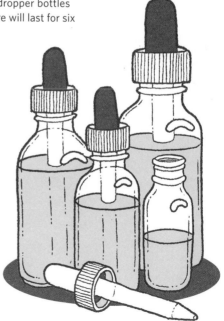

HEMP AS SUPERFOOD

Hemp has nourished people since ancient times, and comes highly recommended by nutritionists as a "perfect" food for humans, since it contains vital proteins edestin and albumin, as well as all eight essential amino acids in the same proportions that our bodies use them. Hemp seed also has the highest concentration of essential fatty acids found in any food on the planet, such as necessary omega-3s and omega-6s that are vital for healthy brain function. Companies like Nutiva, Manitoba Harvest, and Bob's Red Mill market hemp seed as a superfood.

Once a staple ingredient in the porridges of peasants, today slickly packaged hemp cereals, frozen waffles, granola bars, and more crowd the shelves of health food stores, where you can also find hemp seeds, hemp milk, hemp oil, and hemp butter. Here are a few simple suggestions for getting more of this super food into your diet:

- Roast raw hemp seed for a comforting, crunchy, nutty snack similar to roasted pumpkin seeds that can also be sprinkled over popcorn and salads, or mixed into cookie dough, veggie burgers, and oatmeal.

- Hemp oil makes an amazing addition to salad dressings, raw dips like hummus or as a swirl garnishing a bowl of soup. Just don't use hemp oil for sautéing or frying, as high heat will spoil the oil.

- Substitute hemp milk for dairy milk in coffee and smoothies. Or pour it over a nice bowl of hemp granola.

- Hemp butter can be used in baked goods, simple raw desserts, and as a replacement for peanut butter. Try blending hemp butter and almond butter with chopped dates, raisins, hemp seed, walnuts and almonds, plus shredded coconut and powdered cacao to form a basic goo ball that can serve as a quick, energy-dense snack.

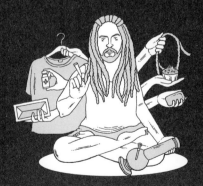

TOPICALS

Cannabis-infused lotions, salves, balms, and other body care products are known collectively as "topicals," which is shorthand for any pot product that's intended for use on the skin. While these modern products are non-psychoactive in low concentrations, they still possess tremendous healing benefits for those with eczema, psoriasis, blemishes, cuts, burns, bruises, other skin conditions, and rheumatoid arthritis. Cannabis-infused lotions and massage oils can also be applied to soothe muscle aches and pains, plus relieve soreness and stiffness. Anyone can benefit from using topicals, since the essential fatty acids contained in cannabis and hemp keep skin and hair supple, smooth, and soft.

Visionary businesspeople are already exploring topicals as a way to increase awareness of the healing properties of cannabis, as well as build a bridge to demographic groups traditionally resistant to drug law reform or marijuana legalization. When a senior citizen learns that a cannabis-infused lotion that won't get him high can still soothe arthritis pain, it changes his perspective on medical marijuana. In Washington state Cannabis Basics and Kush Creams offer full product lines containing everything from lotions and lip balms to medicated tooth picks and tattoo after-care salves; Colorado has Apothecanna; and California's favorite lotion supplier is Doc Green's Healing Collective, which can be found in more than one hundred dispensaries.

Even better, making your own simple cannabis-infused topicals at home couldn't be easier. And after making cannabis-infused lotions, you'll be inspired to create more body care products at home, free from toxic chemicals and harmful synthetic additives. Just think of cannabis products as a "gateway" to a larger world of herbal healing, and a stepping stone to exploring other medicinal herbs like calendula, arnica, tea tree, nettle, and witch hazel. Combining cannabis with other herbs can create healing synergies that beg to be explored.

To get the maximum healing effects from your cannabis, focus on lotions, massage oils, and balms that are absorbed into the skin, not treatments like facial masks or exfoliating scrubs that are rinsed away. Start with this basic recipe, and you'll be feeling the healing in no time!

Basic Cannabis Cream

This fantastic moisturizer and pain-relieving lotion provides relief because the cannabinoids fit into the CB2 receptors in your skin. Store your topicals in an opaque glass container for easy everyday use. Add a nice bow and home-made labels for a thoughtful gift.

MAKES **1** CUP

6 grams cannabis trim (add any stems you might have!)

1¼ ounces almond or grapeseed oil

1½ ounces coconut oil

½ ounce beeswax

1¼ ounces hemp seed oil (from health food store)

4 ounces distilled water

⅓ teaspoon grape-fruit seed extract (preservative)

10 to 25 drops of a fragrant essential oil, if desired

1. Start by infusing your oils with cannabis. Combine the pot with the almond and coconut oils and heat on low in a Crock-Pot for 4 hours, stirring every so often. When you are done with the infusion, strain out the plant material and return oils to the Crock-Pot. Add the beeswax and let it melt. Pour the mixture into a glass bowl and add the water and hemp seed oil. Mix with an electric mixer until thick and creamy. Stir in the grapefruit seed extract and any essential oils you might be using. Scoop a bit into your hand and massage into your skin.

Hemp, Hemp, Hooray!

A GREEN FUTURE

We've already outlined hemp's long and illustrious history, so now let's talk about how hemp can and will help build a sustainable future for the planet.

Once revered for producing fuel, food, medicine, building materials, paper, textiles, and more, this most versatile, completely non-psychoactive plant variety unfortunately got lumped in with marijuana during the original *Reefer Madness* campaign of the 1930s, and as a result, until very recently, American farmers couldn't grow the plant, though food, clothing, soap, and other products made from hemp remained legal.

Now that hemp grows in several states, however, this newly legal domestic supply is already leading to a steep drop in prices for the raw material, spurring serious innovation, and offering an amazing opportunity to replace a wide variety of costly, environmentally damaging products currently made from plastic and petroleum. Hemp can even play an essential role in slowing, stopping, and eventually reversing climate change, creating renewable energy sources and providing the green jobs America needs.

> "Why use up the forests which were centuries in the making and the mines which required ages to lay down, if we can get the equivalent of forest and mineral products in the annual growth of the hemp fields?"
>
> HENRY FORD

THE MODERN HEMP MOVEMENT

The modern hemp movement began in 1985 with the publication of Jack Herer's *The Emperor Wears No Clothes*. By the early 1990s, inspired by this underground book and the man who wrote it, pot activists began tirelessly touting the environmental benefits of hemp while high-minded entrepreneurs built businesses selling clothes, food, and body care products made from the plant.

High Times published a special Earth Day issue dedicated to this amazing natural resource in 1990, then launched a spin-off magazine, *Hemp Times*, and a retail store called Planet Hemp. Influential longtime editor in chief Steven Hager strongly dedicated himself to spreading the word, writing "The truth is legalizing hemp would restructure our national economy and put more money in the hands of American farmers, while devastating the petrochemical industry—the major source of world pollution." Hager also published the writings of Jack Herer to a wide audience, helping to inspire thousands of people to become hemp and cannabis activists.

Determined to revive the hemp industry, Herer delved ever deeper into researching the historical significance and industrial uses of this once vital natural resource. Along the way, he unearthed a copy of *Hemp for Victory*, a 1942 film produced by the U.S. Department of Agriculture urging farmers to grow hemp for the war effort, which he then used as proof of hemp's value. And in a 1990 *High Times* interview, Herer pointed to hemp's potential in combatting the greenhouse effect: "Hemp is the only plant that can completely substitute for fossil fuel. It's an annual that grows in all fifty states and the fastest growing sustainable biomass on the planet."

> **"As for the United States Navy, every battleship requires 34,000 feet of rope. Here in the Boston Navy Yard, where cables for frigates were made long ago, crews are now working night and day making cordage for the fleet.... Hemp for mooring ships; hemp for tow lines; hemp for tackle and gear; hemp for countless naval uses both on ship and shore. Just as in the days when Old Ironsides sailed the seas victorious with her hempen shrouds and hempen sails. Hemp for victory!"**

FROM *HEMP FOR VICTORY*, A 1942 FILM PRODUCED BY THE U.S. DEPARTMENT OF AGRICULTURE

Hemp is helpful here in two ways. First, as a substitute: In 2009, a federally-sponsored report showed that switching from gas to ethanol derived from corn can reduce greenhouse gas emissions by 52 percent, and hemp would prove even more efficient than corn. Second, as a corrective: Climate change happens primarily when the carbon dioxide previously locked into fossil fuels releases into the atmosphere as those fuels are burned to produce heat or energy. As hemp grows, it actually captures CO_2. An acre of hemp, in this way, removes ten times more CO_2 than an acre of trees, while producing quadruple the amount of paper. A hearty crop that requires no harmful pesticides, hemp also improves soil quality when rotated with other plants like canola or soybeans. This is all because hemp's long roots penetrate deep into the ground, aerating the soil and returning biomass, which helps to reverse degrading fertility and erosion—both dire environmental problems.

> "Never give up the ganja."
>
> MORGAN FREEMAN

GOOD AND GOODS FOR YOU

As for durable goods, the possibilities are mind-boggling. Hemp can literally house, clothe, and feed humankind, including as a renewable source of non-polluting fuel, biodegradable plastics, and more!

Hemp's an excellent material for natural building and the construction of eco-friendly, energy-efficient housing. At the University of Bath in England, the BRE Centre for Innovative Construction Materials constructed a small one-story building, called the HemPod on the university campus, monitoring it for temperature and humidity to determine the environmental efficiency of their hemp-lime mixture. As professor Pete Walker, director of the BRE Centre, explained, "Hemp grows so quickly; it only takes the area the size of a rugby pitch to grow enough in three months to build a typical three-bedroom house."

Meanwhile, Hemp Technologies, a sustainable building firm based in North Carolina, is pioneering the use of Hempcrete to construct beautiful homes, including a 3,400 square foot residence for the former mayor of Asheville, dubbed "America's First Hemp House." They estimate this one house has locked in as much carbon dioxide as ten acres of trees,

> "When you smoke the herb, it reveals you to yourself."
>
> BOB MARLEY

while reducing heating and cooling costs by 75 percent. The hemp house also removes the need for toxic building and insulating materials like asbestos, lead, arsenic, and formaldehyde.

Hemp can also replace many plastics currently created from nonrenewable petroleum products. Rather than crowding landfills, polluting the ocean, and poisoning wildlife, "hemplastics" biodegrade, and they're twice as strong as polypropylene. Hemp plastics have already been molded into a wide variety of goods, including DVD cases, digital scales, chairs, and water bottles. JVC even created a speaker cone made from hemp, claiming the plant's "good vibrations" helped sound quality.

Back in the dawn of the automobile era, Henry Ford created a type of resin-stiffened hemp fiber that was ten times stronger than steel, but due to political pressure his prototype hemp cars never rolled off Detroit assembly lines. Fortunately, the idea didn't disappear forever. In 2008, the luxury carmaker Lotus created the Eco Elise, a gorgeous vehicle that uses hemp, eco wool, and sisal extensively throughout its construction. And hemp can not only be used to make cars, it can fuel them too.

Meanwhile, recent advances in hemp-pulping technology now allow for hemp paper to be produced without pollution, and at a lower cost than paper made from wood. Extremely durable hemp paper can also be recycled more times than conventional tree-based paper. Examples of hemp paper more than 1,500 years old have been discovered largely intact.

Textile manufacturing can also return to its roots in hemp by reviving a once thriving trade in durable, beautiful clothing made from the plant. According to the Hemp Industries Association, "hemp fiber is longer, stronger, more absorbent, and more insulative than cotton fiber." Meanwhile, America's cotton fields consume 25 percent of the world's pesticides, while hemp uses none to produce clothing that's lightweight, breathable, soft, and comfortable.

> **"Marijuana refreshes your perspective and allows you to see things in a different way. It's humbled me about my ability to really appreciate things. When you're not high, it reminds you that there might be more to appreciate about something than what you're seeing, hearing, or tasting."**
>
> RICK STEVES

Hemp silks have even been created that can be fashioned into gorgeous wedding dresses, high-end business suits, and other fancy attire. No wonder mainstream apparel brands like Patagonia, Eileen Fisher, Adidas, Calvin Klein, and Ralph Lauren—alongside pioneering smaller hemp clothing companies such as Hemp Works—increasingly feature hemp in some of their products.

GREEN MIND, GREEN BODY

Body care is another major industry where hemp use is poised to grow, as the plant's plentiful essential fatty acids soften skin and hair, replacing ingredients like zinc oxide, butyl stearate, and petroleum laurate for those seeking all-natural, eco-friendly personal care items.

In 1998, visionary businesswoman Anita Roddick launched a line of hemp body care products through her popular Body Shop chain, gaining instant notoriety when French police seized hand cream, lip balm and body butter, claiming the pot leaf posters advertising the line led them to believe cannabis was hiding inside these innocuous tubes and tins.

Another hippie household name, Dr. Bronner's brand of "magic" soaps has famously used hemp oil for years, as pioneered by the company's original founder. Today, his grandson David Bronner is a leading hemp activist who once locked himself in a steel cage outside the White House with a sign proclaiming "Dear Mr. President: Let U.S. farmers grow hemp!" affixed to the top. After a few hours of making his case via bullhorn, the Washington D.C. fire department and police eventually used a chainsaw to cut into the cage and arrest David Bronner. All because our government can't tell the difference between dope and rope!

Certain advocates for hemp have long fought to legitimize their industry by distinguishing hemp from cannabis as two different but related varieties of the same plant. Slogans like "Can't Get High from Hemp" were meant to show consumers that hemp is a serious business, making it easier to reap the environmental benefits of legalizing hemp. The earliest buyers for hemp products were mostly of the "ganja garden variety," however, and so stoking the controversy around marijuana actually helped many of these companies get publicity and market share. So contrary to the strategy of well-meaning activists, it seems that dope ended up helping rope after all.

> **"Some people are just better high."**
>
> JUSTIN TIMBERLAKE

With the passage of state-legal marijuana in Colorado and Washington State, and voters in states such as Vermont, North Dakota, and Kentucky moving to allow commercial hemp, it seems that hemp farming will finally be legitimized as well. Further support has come in the form of a July 2013 report by the Congressional Research Service stating that industrial hemp could be an economically viable option for farmers in a large number of states.

HEMP POWER TO THE PEOPLE!

Now that the power of hemp is about to be unleashed, it's up to consumers to step up and demand not only locally grown fruits and veggies, but locally grown houses, cars and ethanol as well. Such a "re-localization" of necessary commodities and durable goods would revitalize family farming and create thousands, maybe even millions of green jobs, kickstarting a sustainable revolution. Support the hemp movement and help hemp-farming spread across the country by joining activist group Vote Hemp (votehemp.com), and vote with your dollars by purchasing hemp foods, hemp lip balms, hemp coats, and maybe even that Lotus Eco Elise you've always wanted.

The earth will thank you for it!

> "I, as a responsible adult human being, will never concede the power to anyone to regulate my choice of what I put into my body, or where I go with my mind. From the skin inwards is my jurisdiction, is it not? I choose what may or may not cross that border. Here I am the customs agent. I am the coast guard. I am the sole legal and spiritual government of this territory, and only the laws I choose to enact within myself are applicable."
>
> ALEXANDER SHULGIN, BIOCHEMIST AND PHARMACOLOGIST

ACTIVISM:
WHAT CAN I DO?

🌿🌿🌿🌿🌿🌿🌿🌿🌿

Perhaps the only thing that feels better than smoking a nice, fat joint of perfectly grown cannabis is sharing that same joint with some kind-hearted friends after working together to help free the weed. Because, here's the thing, despite all the amazing recent advancements made in marijuana liberation, it's still up to all of us who truly love this plant to keep fighting for our own freedom! So if you haven't already, please start your journey from couchlocked stoner to highly motivated cannabis activist by researching all the wonderful groups already working to end the war on pot, and finding one that's right for you. For all of our forty years, High Times has rolled pretty deep with the National Organization for the Reform of Marijuana Laws (NORML), and so we'd surely suggest starting your journey at norml.org, where you can quickly educate yourself on how to stand up for your rights!

Danko's Best Questions

For years, Danny Danko has been counseling the readers of High Times on picking the right strains, as the author of The Official High Times Field Guide to Marijuana Strains and with his annual "Top 10 Strains" report. Check out this collection of some of the best questions on kinds of cannabis and how to abide by medical-marijuana laws.

WHY ARE SOME STRAINS CLONE-ONLY?

Why can't I get Banana Kush? I've heard of this strain many times, and now I see it's third on your list [of Strongest Strains], which only drives me more insane because we don't have dispensaries in my area and this strain doesn't seem to be available in seed form. So my other question is: Why are some strains clone-only? —*Adam*

Dear Adam,

Some strains are clone-only because the male versions do not exist. They may have popped out of seeds found in a bag of weed or been the result of a particular female phenotype (a rare mutation). Without a reliable male, any crosses made with that plant will reflect only half of the desired genetics, making it tough to stabilize genetics and create a consistent result. Many breeders are working hard to cross back to earlier generations and create seed versions of clone-only varieties, but it's hard work and takes several generations of meticulous crossing and selection.

HOW DO I GET STARTED IN THE CANNABIS INDUSTRY?

This isn't a question on how to grow my medical cannabis, but on how to grow my career in medical cannabis. I want to be involved in the cannabis industry and legalization movement in some capacity; I think I'd like this to be my "career path." My ultimate dream isn't too far off from what you and your producer Mike are doing. To get there, however, I first need to find my start. I have yet to be able to grow due to the high rental prices in this ski town I'm in. I'm moving to a bigger area to deal with this. My question is this: Would moving to Portland, OR, be a bad move when I currently live in Colorado?

My only experience in the industry is from budtending at a local low-volume dispensary, which prompts my second question: Where should I begin? What advice would you give someone who is aspiring to do well in the industry? Is there anything in particular I can do to help my career? Or maybe you could share some piece of advice that helped you do well. —*Jordan*

Dear Jordan,

A career in the cannabis industry and legalization movement isn't for everyone, but I can testify that it's truly as fulfilling as it is fun. Working to free cannabis from prohibition can be challenging, but it helps to know we're on the right side of this fight, and getting to meet and interact with all of the great businesspeople and activists in the movement has been a dream come true.

As for your question: Portland, OR, is a wonderful place with many great opportunities in both the business end and activist end of the movement. Colorado isn't too shabby in that department either, so you should make your decision based on where you'd enjoy living most.

Hopefully, no matter where you end up, you'll have both commerce and activism as a part of your efforts, because all cannabusinesses should be supporting the nonprofits that work to free the plant for everyone, and the only way our fight will be won is if everybody contributes.

My advice for launching your cannabis career is simple: attend as many pot-related events as you can and meet the people that make them happen. The Seattle Hempfest, Boston Freedom Rally, Portland's Hempstalk and the Hash Bash in Ann Arbor, MI, are all great events where you can mingle with people in the industry. Our *High Times* Medical Cannabis Cups and the Cannabis Cup in Amsterdam are also wonderful places to have some fun and learn about the plant and those working to spread the word.

At first, remember to do more listening than talking and absorb everything you can. Learn to discern who knows what they're talking about and who doesn't, and that way you'll be able to separate yourself from the charlatans and shysters who, sadly, infest every burgeoning industry. Above all, work hard and have fun!

ADVICE FOR MY FIRST TRIP TO AMSTERDAM? ↓ I'll be

visiting Amsterdam for three days soon, and I'm looking for advice on what shops to visit and which strains to use. I would like to get out of the main tourist area, but not too far. Also, I don't just want to go there and smoke and not take anything different or positive away from it. I'd like to learn from this special plant.

So my question to you is this: Can you please recommend a coffeeshop to visit with a helpful staff, as well as a *sativa* strain that will give me a cerebral/ spiritual high in the afternoon, followed by an *indica* in the evening to help me relax? —*Thomas*

Dear Thomas,

Amsterdam is a wonderful city for more reasons than one. The coffeeshop scene is amazing, but there are plenty of other things to see as well. As for the coffeeshops, where else in the world can you walk into a comfortable, friendly environment and order cannabis and hashish off a menu and then smoke it at your table, all without a doctor's permission? Some of my favorites are De Dampkring, the Green House, the Grey Area, and Bluebird. You should certainly stop by Barney's for breakfast and try a wonderful *sativa* named Dr. Grinspoon. For an *indica,* get yourself some Shoreline OG from the Green Place. Needless to say, a great time to visit would be in November for our annual *High Times* Cannabis Cup!

Also, be sure to visit the Cannabis College in the red-light district for a comprehensive lesson on marijuana use and activism (you can even take a garden tour). While in the area, stop by Sensi Seeds' Hash, Marijuana and Hemp Museum for a look at the history of our favorite flower. And don't leave the city without visiting the recently reopened Rijksmuseum as well as the Van Gogh Museum. Amsterdam is also home to the greatest number of Vermeer paintings in the world, so be sure to check out some real Dutch masters while you're there.

CAN I GET SEEDS BY MAIL? ⚘ **Hi! I live in the U.S.A. and am 64 years old. Can I buy seeds and have them shipped to me?** —*Wayne*

Dear Wayne,

The seed business is a murky one indeed. Most seed breeders overseas prefer not to ship to the United States, fearing the reach of American prosecutors (and rightly so if you're familiar with the case of Marc Emery, who was extradited to the U.S. from Canada for selling seeds to Americans). This has led to a growing number of retailers or middlemen who purchase wholesale lots of seeds (purportedly from the original breeders) and ship them from countries where the laws against seeds aren't so harsh. The United Kingdom and Spain come to mind as places where this practice has proliferated.

The important thing for you as a purchaser is to do some research on the company and make sure it has a reputation for sending the right seeds and dealing with customer concerns. Steer clear of fly-by-night operations that nobody has heard of and choose a company with years of experience. If I had to name just two, I'd go with Attitude Seeds (cannabis-seeds-bank.co.uk) or Seedsman Seeds (seedsman.com). Both have over ten years of successful transactions under their belts. Good luck!

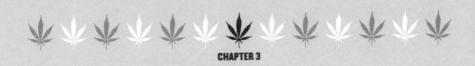

CHAPTER 3

I'm High,

Now What?

DO YOU WANT TO BE

INSIDE

(TURN TO PAGE 176)

or OUTSIDE?

(TURN TO PAGE 178)

I'M NOT SURE . . .

(TURN TO PAGE 180)

INSIDE

NICE . . .
KIND OF MELLOW . . .

- Read a book
- Watch a movie
- Take a nap
- Pet the cat (or dog, ferret . . .)
- Daydream
- Meditate
- Do yoga
- Doodle/draw/paint
- Listen to music
- Dream up new band names
- Stare at the ceiling
- Look at something like you've never seen it before
- Look at old photos
- Drink some tea
- Just chill
- Look at your hands
- Do an easy crossword puzzle
- Play a solitaire card game
- Take a nice warm bath
- Go outside (turn to page 178)

HOW DO YOU FEEL?

AWESOME! ENERGETIC!

- Call a friend
- Play a videogame
- Start a craft project
- Organize something
- Dance around
- Make music
- Write a book
- Write a poem
- Get some work done
- Play dress up
- Make a gravity bong or apple pipe
- Clean your bong
- Take a nice hot/cold shower
- Cook something (turn to page 125)
- Set some goals
- Question authority
- Cut or dye your hair
- Rearrange your bedroom/ living room
- Build a pillow fort
- Go outside (turn to page 178)

OUTSIDE

NICE . . .
KIND OF MELLOW . . .

- Fly a kite
- Close your eyes
- Feel the breeze
- Just listen
- Take a nap
- Watch the clouds
- Watch the stars
- Go to the park
- Go barefoot
- Watch the wildlife
  (birds, squirrels, ducks, the neighbor's cat . . .)
- Watch the sunset
- Count the leaves
- Read a book
- Daydream
- Draw what you see
- Draw what you want to see
- Feel connected to everything
- Stand still
- Watch the grass grow
- Go inside
  (turn to page 176)

HOW DO YOU FEEL?

AWESOME! ENERGETIC!

- Hug a tree
- Climb a tree
- Plant a tree
- Take a hike
- Go for a swim
- Do a cartwheel
- Walk the dog
- Play Frisbee
- Work out
- Make new friends
- Join the circus

- Sing karaoke
- Join the drum circle
- Window shop
- Play tag
- Swing on a swing set
- Roll down a grassy hill
- Jump rope
- Start a pick-up game (soccer, football, volleyball, hacky sack . . .)
- Go inside (turn to page 176)

I'M NOT SURE . . .

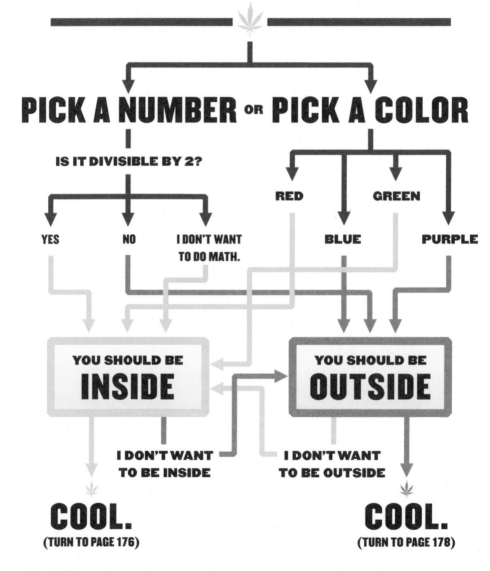

PICK A NUMBER OR PICK A COLOR

IS IT DIVISIBLE BY 2?

YES   NO   I DON'T WANT TO DO MATH.

RED   GREEN   BLUE   PURPLE

YOU SHOULD BE
INSIDE

YOU SHOULD BE
OUTSIDE

I DON'T WANT TO BE INSIDE

I DON'T WANT TO BE OUTSIDE

COOL.
(TURN TO PAGE 176)

COOL.
(TURN TO PAGE 178)

Fun *and* Games

The next time you're hanging with your friends on a quiet night, check out one of these popular herb-smoking games. Designed to encourage creativity and interaction instead of just inebriation, our collection includes physical challenges, strategy sessions, growing and toking challenges, and marijuana-fueled takes on classic drinking games.

THE STONED MILE

PLAYERS

6 or more

YOU WILL NEED

Duct tape

String

1 packed bong and one lighter for each team

Think of Stoned Mile as a relay race that involves passing a bong from one runner to the next like a baton. So first divide up into teams of three or four, then pack a modest sized bong for each team and attach a lighter to it with string and some duct tape. One competitor from each team waits at the starting line, lighter in hand, until the referee yells "Go!" Then they all take a full bong rip, exhale, and race once around whatever track or course you have at hand. Even just around a house or apartment building can be fun!

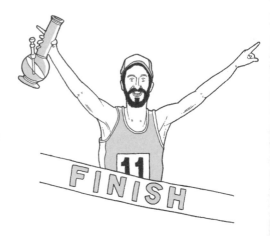

At the completion of one lap, they then hand the bong off to the next member of their team, who promptly takes a bong rip and then runs the same course. Continue until every member of the team has done the same. Anybody who drops the bong, spills the water, empties the bowl accidentally, or loses the lighter merits immediate disqualification. Otherwise, whichever team finishes first wins, provided they smoked the entire bowl.

The prize? More bonghits! ⚬

OUTDOOR GROWER OBSTACLE COURSE

PLAYERS	YOU WILL NEED
unlimited, 1 person runs the course at a time	Stopwatch or timer
	Shovel
	Wheelbarrow
	Several small planting containers
	2 watering cans
	Hose and access to a water source
	3 ten-pound soil bags for each competitor

Cultivating cannabis under the sun is a challenge. Outdoor growers must contend with the elements, as well as wild animals and other pests, while completing physically demanding work each day. So what better way to celebrate the planting of a new pot crop than with an obstacle course designed to train novice growers and apprentices for the rigors of the season? It also adds the thrill of competition to long, boring days spent on the farm, often in remote areas, with little else to do.

Even designing the course offers a lot of fun diversion. Every course will be different, because the terrain and some of the obstacles facing competitors—like haystacks to jump over—will vary based on materials at hand. The course should ideally be a loop, though it can twist and turn depending on the lay of the land. In general, you want something that's grueling but not overwhelming.

One competitor runs the course at a time, with others keeping track of his/her time and watching for penalties. The race begins with a stack of three ten-pound soil bags. The competitor grabs these ten-pound bags, carries them at least twenty yards (sixty feet), and then opens them with a shovel and fills a wheelbarrow with the soil inside. Excessive lost soil will result in a penalty of five minutes added on to a grower's overall time for completing the course.

Next, push the soil-filled wheelbarrow another twenty yards (or more) to a stack of small planting containers and two watering cans. Fill these containers with the soil in the wheelbarrow until the pile disappears (again, five-minute penalty for spilling). Then pick up the watering cans, and race another twenty yards, where you can fill them up with water from a hose. Once they're full, wrap the hose into a coil and sling it over your shoulder. Then it's a mad dash for the finish line, including leaping over a few obstacles en route. And naturally, there's a five-minute penalty for spilling excessively from the watering cans.

Fastest overall time wins, with a prize of sleeping in the next day and skipping morning farm chores! ⚘

BONG BALANCING

PLAYERS

unlimited

YOU WILL NEED

A plastic bong for each contestant

Lightweight household items to pile on top of a bong (optional)

Measuring tape (optional)

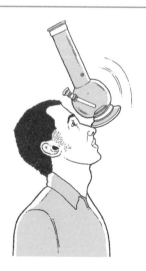

This simple game challenges competitors to carry a plastic bong on top of their heads and walk ten feet. Spilling any water or dropping the bong results in immediate disqualification. Always use a plastic bong full of clean water, as spills will happen.

If balancing a bong on top of your head is too difficult (maybe because you're totally baked), place the bong squarely on the floor or a coffee table, and start to balance household objects on top of it. Gather books, DVDs, empty cups, pinecones, wooden blocks, whatever you might have available. You'll need a measuring tape to record how tall your structures get, then try to beat that record. ✹

TOP TRIMMER

PLAYERS	YOU WILL NEED
unlimited	Stopwatch or timer
	A judge/referee
	1 ounce of untrimmed marijuana and 1 pair of scissors per contestant

Want to prove who's the top trimmer around? What better way than an organized contest to see who can manicure an ounce of pot the fastest? You'll need an impartial judge to assess each trim job, however, as the entire ounce of nugs must be properly tended to with all leaf matter removed from the buds before the clock stops ticking. (See "Bud Trimming Tips," page 90 .) The prize: serious bragging rights, lots of job offers, and a fat sack of herb! ✹

BONG JENGA

PLAYERS	YOU WILL NEED
3 to 6	Jenga set (54 pieces)
	A marker
	A bong and plenty of herb

Take a standard set of Jenga pieces (fifty-four in all), and write the word *bong* on a dozen of them, using the widest side of the wood block. You'll also need 3 to 6 people, a decent amount of herb and a functioning bong to play.

Assemble the Jenga tower as usual. Then, before each turn, each competitor takes a moderate bong rip. If you select a wooden block with the word "bong" on it, you can either take another hit after your turn or "gift" it to a fellow competitor.

Otherwise, standard Jenga rules apply, with each player removing a block and placing it at the top of the tower. Whoever knocks the tower over loses, and must clean the bong and re-pack it for everybody else the entire next round. In the next round, the loser is not allowed to take a hit before every turn, and has to hope he or she gets lucky enough to pull a block that says *bong*. ✹

BONG PONG

PLAYERS	YOU WILL NEED
2 teams	20 cups
	A sturdy table
	Ping-Pong balls
	Plenty of bonghit-sized nuggets (20 for each round)
	A bong for each team

Tired of getting too wasted playing beer pong? Well, here's a safer and healthier variation where inside each of the cups, you'll find a bonghit-sized nugget instead of cheap beer. Just like beer pong, you and your friends will form two teams. Each team places ten cups in a triangle formation on opposite ends of a table, then takes turns throwing ping pong balls into their opponents' cups, taking away a cup and smoking its contents every time they succeed.

To win, eliminate all your opponents' cups first. The prize: Smoking whatever remains in your own. And sticking around to play whoever's next. ⚕

HANDS ON A HALF-OUNCE

PLAYERS	YOU WILL NEED
2 or more, plus a referee	Stopwatch or timer
	A jar filled with herb

This game's exactly like "Hands on a Hard Body"—a contest in Texas where entrants keep their hands on a truck for as long as possible, and whoever lasts the longest wins the truck—only with weed. A competition that will challenge you and your stoner buddies to a brutal endurance test to see who wants a jar of pot the most.

First, fill the jar with an amount of herb that makes sense for you. Naturally, it doesn't really need to be an entire half-ounce, any amount will do, but it should be enough to at least make things interesting (but not enough to create any hard feelings). For a contest amongst growers, or those who have a lot of weight to spare, that might even mean scaling up to a half-pound. You'll just need a much bigger jar! ⚕

The game works best if each contestant contributes an equal amount of herb, or everybody chips in to buy the requisite stash together, but again, whatever works for you. Perhaps one weed-wealthy benefactor will put up the entire amount for the sheer fun of watching his stoner circle square off against one another.

Once the herb's in the jar, place the jar on a table and have each contestant put their fingertips against the glass. When the referee yells the word "Go!", everybody must keep at least four fingers on the jar at all times, with a five-minute break every hour, and a fifteen-minute break every six hours. It's best to appoint one non-participating friend as the referee, charged with timing the breaks and watching out for any accidental hand removal.

Fortunately, each player has one hand free, so you can continue smoking joints. Players can also work to distract others, or try to trick them into removing their hands. No sleeping allowed, so make sure to smoke mostly sativas. The official hardbody truck contest once lasted seventy-seven continuous hours, so let's see if stoners love pot as much as Texans love trucks! ⚘

DRUG WAR

PLAYERS	YOU WILL NEED
2	1 deck of cards
	A joint and a backup joint

This variation on the classic card game War involves smoking a large joint as two players draw from a deck of cards. Prepare a backup joint in case the first is completely smoked before the game ends. Like the real drug war, this game can go on indefinitely.

While one player rolls the joints, the other should shuffle and deal out cards from a standard deck one at a time, alternately, until each player holds half, face down. Then light the joint.

To start, both players take the card off the top of their deck and slap it on the table at the same time, revealing its value. Whoever has the higher card hits the joint, and takes the two cards, returning them to the bottom of his or her deck. When cards of equal value are drawn, it's time for a "drug war," and players draw three cards each and lay them face down on the table. Then each produces a fourth card, face-up, to determine the winner, who is rewarded with all ten cards. If a player who has lost a war checks his or her own three downward-facing cards and finds among them a 4 and a 2 of any suit, the player then wins that war.

The ultimate winner of the game is the incredibly stoned person holding all the cards at the end! ⚕

STONER CHESS

PLAYERS	YOU WILL NEED
2	Materials to make a DIY stoner chess set (32 total)
	Colored paper or cloth to construct a large chessboard
	Herb to smoke from each piece

Taking inspiration from the incredible pieces of smokeable glass pipe art available, a group of enterprising stoners can assemble a set of DIY/scavenged stoner chess pieces and make their own unique addition to the project.

Enlist your friends to collect as many different pieces of glass paraphernalia as possible. You'll need (for example) sixteen one-hitters or spoons to use as pawns, four chillums to serve as rooks, four sidecars as knights, four hammers as bishops, two smaller bongs to be the queens and two larger bongs to be the kings. Choose pieces with similar colors to make two opposing sets, or mark the pieces with stickers to distinguish them.

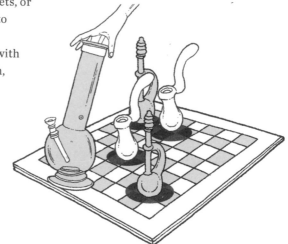

Create a large chessboard with pieces of colored paper or cloth, with each square measuring about two square feet, and set it up on the floor in a large room. Play chess as usual, except you must smoke from each piece in order to move it. Guaranteed to lead to some interesting checkmates! ⚕

ZONK

PLAYERS

2 to 6

YOU WILL NEED

Six colored dice (preferably two red, two white, and two green)

A bong

A decent amount of herb (at least an ounce)

A sheet of paper for keeping score

An elaborate and entertaining dice game, Zonk was created in a freshman dorm in the late 1970s somewhere in upstate New York. Players earn points (and bonghits!) by rolling six dice during each turn.

Each player is first assigned a special nickname, decided upon by the other players. During the game, you can only refer to the person by that special nickname—failure to do so will result in a Zonk (loss of all points) and a skipped turn for the offender. To keep score, write the nicknames across the top of a sheet of paper in the order of the person's turn, and tally the points earned below each name, keeping a running total. If someone zonks, then record a "Z."

Begin by having each player roll a die to determine order of play, with highest roll going first (reroll among players tying for high number until one prevails). Play order will then proceed clockwise from the high roller.

Each turn begins with rolling all six dice, and can end in one of two ways: by choosing to stop and keep your points, or by "zonking out" with no points.

A player wins by being the first to score 5,000 points. Scoring is based on rolling 1s, 5s, and three-of-a-kinds, which is called a "trip." A Zonk occurs when the roll of the dice returns no 1s, 5s, or three-of-a-kinds.

Rolling a 1 is worth 100 points, and a 5 is worth 50 points. A "trip" is worth the value of the number rolled times 100, so triple-3s would be worth 300 points, and a triple-5 would be worth 500 points. An exception is triple-1s, which are worth 1000 points.

After each roll, you must choose between keeping scoring dice or continuing to roll them. For example, if you rolled six dice and yielded a 1-3-3-3-5-6, you could choose to keep the triple 3s (worth 300 points), the 1 (worth 100 points), and the 5 (worth 50 points) or any combination of them. Whatever dice you'd like to keep are set aside, and you continue rolling with the rest. Suppose you decide to keep the triple 3 and the 1 (totaling 400 points), and continue rolling with the 5 and 6. If those two dice return a 2 and a 3, then

NAME	FALCONSMOKER	BIFFY	GIGANTOR	SACKO
ROLL 1	300	Z	50	150
ROLL 2	Z	Z	300	1000
ROLL 3	150	Z*	Z	1300
ROLL 4	850*	150	Z	2000*
ROLL 5	2000*	500*	150	Z

FIG. 1: SAMPLE ZONK SCORESHEET
Marks when a player has earned a Bonghit (BH)

you've zonked, lost all of your points, and your turn is over. If those two dice return with two 1s, then you can choose to keep them and the additional 200 points for a total of 600. Or, you can choose to roll all six dice again, losing the 400 points you've already accumulated to order to try again and potentially score higher. A player who scores on their first roll must keep at least one of them. So if you rolled 1-6-6-3-6-6, you must choose either the 1, the triple-6s, or the combination of the triple-6s and the 1.

If all six dice have returned a score, including dice in play and your previously kept dice, then you set aside all the dice, record the points you've scored, and roll all six dice again. So if you roll a 1-1-1-4-3-5 and you keep the trip 1s, for a running total of 1000, then roll the 4-3-5 again and return a 1-5-5, then all six dice are "scoring dice." Tally up the 1,200 points and roll again.

You may stop your turn and keep the accumulated points (and bonghits! See below) only when four or five dice are scoring dice. So if your roll returns 5-5-5-1-6-4, you can keep the triple 5s for 500 points and the 1 for 100 points, and choose to end your turn with 600 points earned.

A player needs to keep at least 500 points on his or her first roll to "Get in The Game" and earn the first automatic bonghit (BH). Automatic BHs are retained, whereas a Conditional Bonghit can be lost if a player zonks out. On each turn after the first, a player must keep rolling until earning at least 300 points, or until zonking.

There are also several special scoring combinations that earn a player bonghits and extra points. These are as follows:

- **Trainwreck:** This is a major Zonk, occurring when all six dice are rolled at the same time and return all non-scoring integers. For example, if your roll returned 2-2-3-3-4-6, then you've been "trainwrecked," and your consolation prize is an automatic BH.

- **Royale:** A six-dice-straight is called a "royale," and happens when rolling all six dice at once yields 1-2-3-4-5-6. A royale earns 1,500 points and two bonghits—one automatic and one conditional. Plus, since a royale is composed of all "scoring dice," the player must roll again and add the 1,500 points to his or her total.

- **Colors:** If a trip is rolled with one of each color die, then you earn a conditional BH. To illustrate, if a 4-4-4 combination is rolled with one white, one red and one green die, then you get an extra bonghit, provided you don't zonk out before the end of your turn.

- **Nicely Done:** If all six dice are played one at a time, eventually resulting in all six dice being scoring dice, then this is referred to as "nicely done," and earns the player a conditional BH. So, you would start by rolling all six dice, and keep only one 1 or 5 and roll the remaining five dice again. If that roll yielded at least one 1 or 5, then you'd keep that and roll the remaining 4 dice, and so on until only 1s and 5s remained. Since these are all scoring dice, the player would record the points and the conditional BH and roll all six dice again for a "continuation."

Additionally, for each 1,000 points scored in one turn, an automatic BH is earned. If a player zonks three times in a row, earning no points and no BHs, then an automatic BH is granted. If a player scores over 5,000 points, then another automatic BH is added to the tally.

The game is considered over when any player reaches 5,000 points or more during a turn. However, during this "last round," every other player gets a chance at one final turn to attempt to beat the high score. On their last turn, players must continue rolling until they either zonk, or stop their turn with a scoring total higher that the previous record-holder. No player can choose to stop their turn until four or five dice are scoring dice.

At the end of the last round, the player with the most points is the winner, who enjoys the reward of an enormous bonghit. A consolation BH is given to whichever player earned the fewest bonghits during the game.

Additional variations to gameplay and more details on rules can be found online at zonkthegame.com. ⚘

Acknowledgments

To my husband David Bienenstock, for everything.

I'd like to thank all of my cannabis colleagues in the marijuana movement, especially the staff, management and contributors at *High Times* magazine, whose 40-year fight to legitimize cannabis use is finally coming to fruition. I'd especially like to thank *High Times* publisher Mary McEvoy for her confidence in my talents, as well as Michael and Eleanora Kennedy, Judy and Cathy Baker, and Colleen and Jessica Manley for keeping the legacy of Tom Forçade alive!

Richard Cusick, Danny Danko, Bobby Black, Nico Escondido, and Dan Skye all write regularly for *High Times*, and contributed their writing and expertise directly to *Marijuana for Everybody!*

I'm especially grateful to all of the pot pioneers profiled in this book, including Jack Herer, Valerie Corral, Dr. Lester Grinspoon, Martin A. Lee, Fred Gardner, Mila Jansen, Robert Connell Clark, Michael & Michelle Aldrich, Chris Bennett, Larry "Ratso" Sloman, Mason Tvert, Clint Werner, Professor Robert Melamede, Dr. Sanjay Gupta, Dr. Mitch Earlywine, Bob Snodgrass, Eagle Bill, and David Bronner. Other important contributors to this book include Ed Murrieta, Chris Lanter, Portland's Skunk Pharm Crew, Kym Kemp, and our favorite photographer Lochfoot with his Cali Cannons.

And to my new friends on the West Coast, including California NORML, especially Dale Gieringer and Ellen Komp, everyone at the Multidisciplinary Association for Psychedelic Studies including Brian Brown, Kynthia Brunette, Brad Burge, Colin Hennigan, and Berra Yazar-Klosinski; the fine folks at WAMM and David Downs at the *East Bay Express*, thank you for your kindness and commitment to ending cannabis prohibition.

And to the *High Times* Cannabis Cup crew, for their hard work and camaraderie. Including Thumpah Lee and Sean Black who offered technical advice for this book.

This book owes its life to the consistent efforts of Steve Mockus, Emily Dubin, Lia Brown, Michelle Clair, Courtney Drew, and my awesome agent, Alex Glass at Trident Media Group. And a big thank-you to Toby Triumph for the wonderful illustrations.

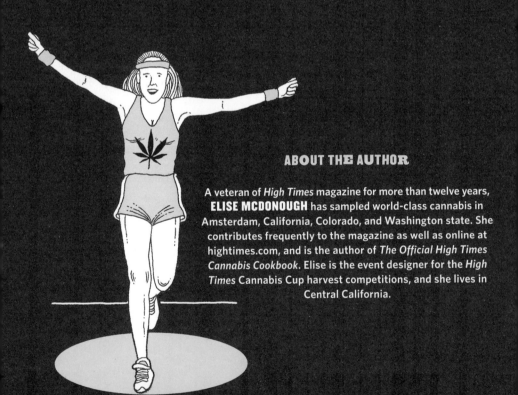

ABOUT THE AUTHOR

A veteran of *High Times* magazine for more than twelve years, **ELISE MCDONOUGH** has sampled world-class cannabis in Amsterdam, California, Colorado, and Washington state. She contributes frequently to the magazine as well as online at hightimes.com, and is the author of *The Official High Times Cannabis Cookbook*. Elise is the event designer for the *High Times* Cannabis Cup harvest competitions, and she lives in Central California.